# The Soul of the Caring Nurse:
## Stories and Resources for Revitalizing Professional Passion

Linda Gambee Henry
and James Douglas Henry

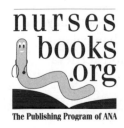

nurses
books
.org

The Publishing Program of ANA

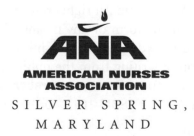

AMERICAN NURSES
ASSOCIATION

SILVER SPRING,
MARYLAND

Library of Congress Cataloging-in-Publication Data

Henry, Linda Gambee.
  The soul of the caring nurse: stories and resources for revitalizing professional passion / by Linda Gambee Henry and James Douglas Henry.
    p. ; cm.
  Includes bibliographical references.
  ISBN 1-55810-219-1
  1.  Nursing--Philosophy. 2.  Nursing--Anecdotes. 3. Caring. 4. Nursing--Practice.
  [DNLM: 1.  Nurses--psychology--Personal Narratives. 2.  Attitude of Health Personnel--Personal Narratives. 3.  Job Satisfaction--Personal Narratives. WY 100 H522s 2004]  I. Henry, James Douglas. II. Title.

  RT84.5.H465 2004
  610.73--dc22

                          2004006266

Published by
Nursesbooks.org
The Publishing Program of ANA
American Nurses Association
8515 Georgia Avenue
Suite 400
Silver Spring, MD 20910-3492
http://www.nursingworld.org

*Book design and composition*
House of Equations, Inc., Hanover, NH

*Cover design*
Stacy Maguire, Eyedea Advertising
  & Design Studio, Sterling, VA

*Printing and manufacturing*
McArdle Printing, Upper Marlboro, MD

First printing April 2004. Second printing September 2006.
ISBN-13: 978-1-55810-219-4      ISBN-10: 1-55810-219-1      SAN: 851-3481

04SCN      2.5M      09/06R

## Dedication

We dedicate this book with profound gratitude to nurses everywhere and especially to all the nurses who enthusiastically agreed to be interviewed. We are honored by their trust. We are moved by their passion and commitment to the profession and to making a difference in people's lives. Our heartfelt thank you.

# Contents

**Acknowledgments**  *ix*

**Introduction**  *xi*

**Using this Book**  *xxx*

**About the Authors**  *xix*

*Part I   Nurses Stories From the Heart*  1

MIDWIFE AT THE EXIT  3
Christine Hall, BA, RN, CHPN
*Wounded healer who paints her patients*

JOE'S MOM—A STORY OF TRANSFORMATION  7
Lisa M. Wayman, MSN, RN
*ICU nurse: A mother's pain, a professional's passion*

DANCING WITH THE ATOMS IN THE UNIVERSE  11
Deborah McElligott, RN, ANP, HNP
*Holistic nurse practitioner: Visionary with a healing plan*

TENACITY WITH A SMILE  15
Steven H. Brant, BSN, RN, PHN
*Navy nurse: Committed optimist*

GIVING SMALL GIFTS  19
Janet E. Hersh, RN, CNICU, CCRN
*ICU nurse: Empathy and imagination*

EMPOWERING PRESENCE OF HEART   23
Diane M. Newman, BSN, RN
*Cardiac nurse: Work as a kind of love*

COMPASSIONATE CATALYST   27
Susan Huntley, RN
*Clinic Nurse: Enabling energy to flow*

FELLOW SOJOURNER   31
Joan E. Purdon, MSN, CS, RN
*Parish nurse: Nursing spirituality*

I CAN DO THAT!   35
Dee Lowe Horn, RN
*Home care nurse: Enterprising up-front organizer*

CONNECTING THROUGH COMPETENCE AND COMPASSION   39
Carolyn Spence Cagle, PhD, RNC
*Nursing professor: Change agent*

ANYTHING'S POSSIBLE   43
Sister Peggy Fannon, RSM, RN, CDE
*Merciful patient educator*

ADVOCATE AT THE END OF LIFE   47
Eve-lynn Civerolo, RN
*Hospice nurse: Passion for helping others pass on*

LET'S GET BUSY! LOOKING FOR THE POSSIBLE   52
John Hanson, BS, RN
*Former Traveling Nurse: 23 countries, 32 states, 8 years*

WE'LL GET THERE!   55
Karen D. Beatty, MSN, RN, BSN
*Visiting nurse: African American PIPE queen*

NURSING IN THE FOXHOLE   58
Amy Brown, BSN, RN
*Psychiatric nurse: Unconditional positive regard*

HAVE A PLAN   62
Bettina Pangan, BSN, RN
*Clinical analyst seeing both sides of care*

SOCIAL NURSE-A-WORKER   66
Marianne Davis, RN
*Legendary strategist: Piloting people through the healthcare maze*

PASSIONATE TENACITY   70
Naomi Mason, BSN, RN, PHN
*Native American Shoshone obstacle remover*

CARING WITH A DISCERNING EYE   74
Sandi Harding, MA, RN
*Parish nurse: Hugs and blessings*

*Part II   Strategies for Organizational and Individual Caring   79*

**Creating Healthy, Caring Organizational Culture—Strategies and Resources   81**

    The Role of Leadership   82
        A New Facility, A New Culture: Harrison Memorial Hospital   82
        Core Leadership Competencies: Baptist Health Care   83

    Education and Staff Development   86
        Compassionate Communication: Harrison Memorial Hospital   86
        Cost Savings Through Staff Care: MultiCare Regional Cancer Center   87
        Reigniting Nursing Passion: Colleen Person   90
        Nominal Group Technique: Inge Christensen   92

    Models for Caring   93
        A Magnet Facility: University of Colorado Hospital   93
        A Planetree Affiliate Facility: Longmont United Hospital   96
        The Caring Model™: Sharon Dingman's Synthesis of Caring Theories   98

**Caring for Your Nursing Career   103**

        Parental Influence on Careers   105
        Rearview Mirror Exercise   106
        Establish and Participate in a Speaking Event   106
        Pay Attention to Your Words   107
        Pay Attention to Your Body   107
        Talk to Your Guardian Angel   108
        Take Yourself to the Bookstore   108
        Whose Job Do You Want?   108

    Two Instruments, One Goal: Finding the Gifts of You   108
        Skill Clusters Inventory   109
        Instructions   110
        Transferable Skills Card Sort   110
        Nursing Career Interests   112

**Strategies and Resources for Nurse Self-Care   115**

        Connect to Community   115
        Build Healthy Relationships   115

Share Your Story and Listen to the Stories of Others    117
     OH Cards    117
     A PBS Home Video on Everyday Spirituality    117
     A Book of Storytelling Starters    117
     A Book for Work Groups    118
     Some Internet Sites    118
     This Book    118
Call a Circle    118
Visit the "Nurses Are Angels" Web Site    118
Focus upon Possibilities, Not Problems    118
Explore the Expectations of Others and Communicate Your Expectations    119
Practice Appreciative Inquiry    119
Live Your Life with Intentionality    119
Anchor Yourself in the Present Moment    119
Care Enough Not to Actively Care    120
Practice the Art of Human Complexity    120
Laugh and Engage Humor    120
Live with Open-Ended Questions    121
Pray    121
Practice Meditation    122
Live Simply    122
Practice Forgiveness    122
Prepare Food and Eat Soulfully    123
Connect with Nature    123
Exercise    123
Join the International Association for Human Caring (IAHC)    123
Join the Relationship-Centered Care Network    124
Participate in the Nurse Manifest Network    124
Explore Holistic Nursing    124
Take a Vow-of-Kindness Pledge    124
Give Yourself a Sabbath Day    125
Listen    125
Listen to Music    126
Complete the Self-Care Audit    126
Develop a Self-Care Plan    127

Reflections on Caring: The Cycle of Self and Others    128

**Appendix, Sample of Interview Questions    131**

**Notes    133**

# Acknowledgments

We greatly appreciate the many people who made this book possible. To the nurses who so graciously allowed us to capture their stories, the nurse executives and managers who shared strategies for self-care, the caring for others and building caring environments, all of the people who so enthusiastically supported this work and pointed us to additional resources, the willingness of the ANA to endorse a "different" kind of publication and to our editor Eric Wurzbacher for his continued support and creativity, our heartfelt thanks.

Both we and the publisher are deeply grateful as well to the reviewers of the original manuscript and/or the initial book proposal. They are: Tamara Cyhan, RN, BSN, Member of the Publishing Advisory Board of nursesbooks.org; Bonnie Faherty, PhD, APRN-BC, Cm, Healthcare consultant in private practice and emeriti faculty member, Department of Health Sciences, California State University Northridge (CSUN); Patricia D. Kissell, PhD, RN, Chair, Department of Nursing, Northwest Nazarene University; Gayle Newshan, PhD, NP, RN, CS; Department of Holistic Care, St. John's Riverside Hospital, Yonkers, NY; Marylee Pakieser MSN, RN, FNP, Michigan Nurses Association; Jackie R. Pfeifer, RN, CCRN, Staff Nurse, Cardiac Center of Luther Hospital, Midelfort Clinic, Eau Claire, WI; and Jane C. Rothrock, DNSc, RN, CNOR, FAAN, Director, Perioperative Programs, Delaware County Community College, Media, PA. In addition, we thank another reviewer, Carol Kenner, DNS, RNC, FAAN, Dean, School of Nursing, University of Oklahoma, for her contribution.

Finally, our gratitude to the nurses who so warmly endorsed this work: Sonja Simpson RN, MSN, HNC, President, American Holistic Nurses Association; Gwen Sherwood, RN, PhD, FAAN, Professor and Executive Associate Dean, The University of Texas Health Science Center at Houston School of Nursing and President-Elect, International Association for Human Caring; and Jean Watson, PhD, RN, FAAN, HNC, Distinguished Professor of Nursing, Chair of Caring Science, University of Colorado Health Sciences Center.

# Introduction

**Anyway**

*People are unreasonable, illogical, self-centered*
*Love them anyway*
*If you do good, people will accuse you of selfish ulterior motives*
*Do good anyway*
*If you are successful, you win false friends and true enemies*
*Succeed anyway*
*The good you do today may be forgotten tomorrow*
*Do good anyway*
*Honesty and frankness will make you vulnerable*
*But be honest and frank anyway*
*People love underdogs, but follow only topdogs*
*Follow some underdogs anyway*
*People really need help, but may attack you if you help them*
*Help people anyway*
*Give the world the best that you have and you may get kicked in the*
*Teeth*
*But give the world the best you have anyway.*

—Author unknown
Found hanging in the lobby of one of the
orphanages where Mother Teresa ministered

*"Science and technology are the palate and paint of the profession;*
*nurses are the artists of healing."*

—An RN

We began *The Soul of the Caring Nurse* with the desire to capture the extraordinary stories of some ordinary nurses, to present their chronicles that hopefully will build bridges of understanding and will inspire other nurses to revitalize their own passion for the profession, affirming a sense of "That's why I'm a nurse." We interviewed almost 30 nurses for this book, some of whom shared how they transitioned from burnout to reach a time of revitalized self-assurance, purpose, and passion in their nursing careers. We also captured more than 100 strategies, resources, and tools for personal, patient, and organizational caring.

Many nurses enter the profession with a profound sense of calling, a desire to care for others and to make a difference in people's lives at their most vulnerable times. "The soul of caring," notes Tina Pangan, RN (whose story you will read later in this book), "is the ability to share oneself in a sincere and loving manner. Nursing is a profession that allows us to give another human being a piece of ourselves without fear of judgment. Nursing is a great profession because it connects you with people!"

Stress and the ongoing changes present in today's healthcare arena can overshadow the initial sense of calling and may lead to a sense of career disenchantment and feelings of burnout. It is one of the reasons why the American Nurses Association's Code of Ethics for Nurses underscores the importance of meaningful work and self-care in the fifth of its nine ethical provisions:

> The nurse owes the same duties to self as to others, including the responsibility to preserve integrity and safety, to maintain competence and to continue personal and professional growth.[1]

It goes without saying that, today, health care in general is in need of significant reform. As a discipline, we believe that the nursing profession often leads the way in this respect, advocating a holistic approach to health care and healing. Many nurses view body, mind, emotion, and spirit as being interconnected in terms of their impact upon healing. While the holistic nature of nursing is self-evident to any practicing nurse or a nurse's patient or client, this quality is also recognized in the 2004 publication that establishes the essentials of nursing practice. "The nursing needs of human beings are identified from a holistic perspective and are met within the context of a culturally sensitive, caring interpersonal relationship. . . . Nursing embraces dynamic processes that affect the human person, including . . . spirituality, healing, empathy, mutual respect, and compassion. These intangible aspects foster health."[2]

Additionally, there is a growing body of ongoing research into the nature and processes of caring and healing that are implemented across a wide range of practices. Since 1992, for instance, the National Center for Complementary and Alternative Medicine (NCCAM) of the National Institutes of Health has been exploring complementary and alternative healing practices in terms of rigorous science, as well as training complementary and alternative researchers and disseminating to the public and healthcare professionals their findings and related authoritative information.

We will also provide a wealth of strategies, resources, and tools gathered from our interviews with nurses and from a variety of other sources. By dipping into this resource guide, we hope and trust that nurses will become reenergized in their current work environments or in other healthcare arenas. In addition, it is hoped that nursing schools and healthcare organizations will assist nurses and other providers to more completely identify and utilize their key talents and skills as they provide patient care, creating a more soulful environment.

Colleen Person, BSN, RN, MMA, Vice President of Creative Health Care Management, has nearly 40 years' experience in nursing and today finds great joy in facilitating workshops that are designed to reignite passion for caring relationships. "In the 1980s and 1990s, we became so preoccupied with the technological aspects of nursing that we lost sight of some of this interconnection," she believes. "And we lost sight of nursing's original calling and commitment so well represented by Florence Nightingale. I believe nursing stands as a rather unique profession in that the heart of it is relationship. No one else provides such a bio/psycho/social/spiritual service, but we became caught up in the biological dimension for a period of time with its emphasis upon the medical/technical model. We lost our soul and our relationship with patients as the reason for being.

"In addition, in the mid-1990s, we got caught up in the accountant-based redesign of health care, or to use a recently coined term, the 'Enronization' of nursing. Financial considerations became the reason for restructuring, and much of the activity involved doing something *to* nursing instead of *with* nursing, further demoralizing the profession. Many nurses experienced a profound amount of emotional pain.

"However," she continues, "by way of a more proactive leadership and through the pioneering work of nurses such as Jean Watson, Kristen Swanson, Madeleine Leininger, Sharon Dingman, and others, a reformation began to take place.[3] In particular, Jean Watson gave voice to nurses being called to special therapeutic and healing relationships with patients at some of the most challenging moments in their lives."

"With relationship-based care, the nurse as primary caregiver knows a person's story, not only the current situation, but how it fits into other chapters of the person's life. It refocuses task-based care to needs-based care within the context of person-to-person relationships. At the same time, it underlines the importance of having a theory as a framework for care. So, beginning in the late 1990s, we began to see organizations adopting and adapting the work of Watson, Swanson, Dingman, and others, or they were developing a model of their own."

Today, Colleen asserts that nurses, like the phoenix, are beginning to rise from the ashes of the past to reclaim their unique professional caring relationships with patients and with one another, not only in the context of theory, but also in that of a care delivery model. Such a model organizes how the relationship and activities of care will be accomplished within clinical specialties maximizing the mix of staff and other resources.

Colleen suggests that one of the first steps paramount in developing a nursing theory and a nursing care delivery model for their organization is to assist nurses to reconnect with their original sense of calling and to engage with proactive creativity in order to make a difference in health care. "Last year I attended an international congress of nursing and was struck by the commonality of values and problems throughout the world, as well as innovative strategies for reigniting the flame that Florence Nightingale carried among the pallets of the soldiers."

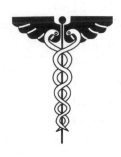

Reconnecting with this sense of calling is not only vital for the individual nurse, but we believe remains critical to the reformation of health care in general. In his book *The Way of the Physician,*[4] philosopher, historian, and prolific writer Jacob Needleman (1985) brings to light the fact that there are two serpents rather than one in most images of the caduceus, which is widely accepted as the emblem of medicine. He suggests that the two serpents represent two fundamental energies. The more left-brain energy focuses upon rational, analytical, and technical exploration and competence.

It serves as the "doing" aspect of health care. Its opposite force concentrates attention upon "being." It is relational and concerned with compassionate caring. Both of these energies apply equally to health care and healing; one without the other leaves the system crippled.

Needleman believes that the orientation of most healthcare professionals in today's technological, competitive, and results-oriented environment is unfortunately one-sided. Health care relies heavily upon clinical investigation and application. Even the caduceus displayed by the American Medical Association contains only one serpent. So, where are we to turn for balance to embrace "being" and to experience compassionate health care? Fortunately, there exists an accelerating movement to restore balance as exemplified by organizations such as Fetzer Institute's Relationship Centered Care Network, Magnet hospitals, and Planetree affiliates, all of which promote patient-centered care and people-friendly healing environments.[5] However, we believe that today the most concentrated, cutting edge transformative activities are occurring in the *profession of nursing*, especially as it returns to its historic roots of holistic health care.

This book is about nurses, their stories, tragedies, and triumphs. It is also about nurse leaders who seek to create healthy, caring work environments. And it is hoped nurses and lay people alike will find it helpful as a resource guide of strategies to enhance the caring of self and others.

We particularly called the attention of the nurses we interviewed to the research of Kristen Swanson, PhD, RN (1991) and her five processes of caring because they are especially easy to understand and apply.[6]

Kay Lanier, RN, BSN, MA, Clinical and Operations Director at the MultiCare Regional Cancer Center in Tacoma, Washington, brought Kristen Swanson in-house for a day of education with all the unit's nurses. With Kristen's permission, they subsequently adapted the five processes to support the unit's philosophy and environment, as the following page shows, with just a few examples for each process.

| Processes of Caring Kristen Swanson, PhD, RN | Description |
|---|---|
| **Maintaining Belief** | The foundation for caring. Believing that there is meaning to be found in the situation. Maintaining hope in long-term healing. Going the distance ("I'm in this with you"). |
| **Knowing** | Striving to understand the event as it has meaning in the life of the other. Thoroughly assessing the condition. Centering on the one cared for. Avoiding assumptions. |
| **Being With** | Conveying availability and ability. Listening and giving feedback on what is said or felt. Conveying that the person's experience matters. Caring without burdening oneself. |
| **Doing For** | Doing for others what they would do for themselves if they could. Anticipating and performing competently. Preserving the dignity of the person. |
| **Enabling** | Enabling others to practice self-care. Providing information and explaining. Helping to generate alternatives and providing feedback. |

Behaviors such as those below are evaluated on an almost daily basis simply by listening and observing nurses as they go about their work. Kay also maintains that rarely does she hear a nurse using impersonal language, such as "the disruptive patient in Room Three." Rather, each patient is seen as a human soul to be cared for and not judged, regardless of things such as temperament, age, addictive behaviors, ethnic background, or social status.

We divided this book into two parts. The first part contains stories of nurses, while the second part collects the strategies for organizational and individual caring for other nurses.

In Part I, the stories of the nurses we interviewed are not meant to be representative of the nursing profession as a whole, we attempted to select nurses in as diverse

| Processes | Behaviors |
|---|---|
| **Being Present** | ▪ Centering on the person cared for, not thinking of another patient as a new room is entered<br>▪ Avoiding assumptions by checking with the patient and family about their meanings of illness and healing |
| **Being Open** | ▪ Honoring the patient's right to decide what to do, wear, or eat or how to sleep or bathe<br>▪ Sharing feelings without burdening patient and family |
| **Being Competent** | ▪ Promoting shared problem solving using the team approach with patient and family, nurses, physician, PT/OT, dietary counselor, oncology counselor, CNS, etc.<br>▪ Providing personal privacy and maintaining confidentiality |
| **Being Supportive** | ▪ Teaching self-care strategies<br>▪ Offering positive distractions such as humor, library, family room, quiet room, individual Walkman with selection of tapes, CDs, videos |
| **Being Respectful** | ▪ Displaying esteem for the patient and family belief system<br>▪ Maintaining a hope-filled attitude that offers realistic optimism expressed in the nurse's attitude, language, and actions |

specialties and geographic locations as possible: Every nurse should find something useful from most if not all of these stories. We identified those we interviewed in a variety of ways, including the personal suggestions of nursing executives and nurses, recommendations of healthcare organizations located in areas where we conducted conference presentations and workshops, and among the participants attending an International Association for Human Caring conference, 95% of whom were nurses. A list of interview questions was given to each person prior to our visit, as reported in the Appendix. We did not use all of them with each interviewee, but allowed the discussion to evolve and flow as deemed appropriate. Almost all the interviews were conducted in person, tape-recorded, transcribed, and in some situations, expanded through research.

We incorporated a methodology called *action research*, a spiral process that alternates between action (in our case, interviewing), critical reflection, and research. (Action research is a type of applied research that focuses on innovation and change. Applied research itself, being concerned with developing practical approaches to resolve a given problem, with such approaches based on the knowledge generated by an investigation. While applied research is usually less generalizable than basic research because of this problem-specific orientation, these two research approaches tend to be complementary.)[7]

Several of the stories reflect particular religious orientations. However, it is not our intent to link the nursing profession, or the nature and processes of caring, to any specific spiritual tradition.

Each person also completed two instruments, the Skill Clusters Inventory and the Transferable Skills Card Sort, which are included on pages 108–12 toward the end of the section entitled Caring for Your Nursing Career. We then explored how her or his key skills apply to Swanson's five processes of caring because they are especially easy to understand and apply. We sought to identify an overall theme for each nurse, which became the title for his or her chapter.

For example, "I Can Do That" serves as a theme for enterprising nurse Dee Horn. Dee utilizes all five of the caring processes in her work, but especially excels at enabling others to practice self-care. Hospice nurse Eve-lynn Civerolo cares deeply about allowing her patients to control how they wish to pass on and is an "Advocate at the End of Life." Such themes serve as a unifying and engaging sense of career direction and life/work purpose for these individuals.

We also explored the meaning of soul during these interviews, asking several of the nurses to share perceptions of its importance. Though the soul is mysterious and beyond definition, we nevertheless uncovered a general consensus. For example, cardiac nurse Diane Newman reports, "Soul represents the spiritual essence of a person." Staff nurse Sue Huntley states, "If you had asked me that 20 years ago, I would have a different answer. To me, soul was what we humans had. Other creatures and things did not have a soul. However, today my understanding is that everything has a soul. I identify life energy with soul."

We continue to report nurse stories in Part II, but with an emphasis upon how nurse executives and other healthcare leaders build healthy, caring work environments. It includes an interview at a Magnet hospital (certified by the American Nurses Credentialing Center as providing a positive, supportive environment for nurses), at a Planetree facility (again, certifying excellence in nurse and patient care), and one organization listed as a Fortune 100 Best Employer. Part II also includes a section on caring for and enhancing your nursing career. It concludes with a segment offering over 35 general strategies for personal self-care and caring for others.

Arguably, the working environment of nurses today is fraught with many obstacles, from managed care and dwindling resources to staffing shortages. Some people suggest that such barriers prevent nurses from caring for their patients in the ways they might like. This book is not about fixing the system. The reality, as John Hanson, RN, sees it, is that, "There will always be something in the system that needs changing—that prevents us from practicing nursing as we might like." Rather, *The Soul of the Caring Nurse* offers a perspective on how nurses can and do practice caring *in spite of* the current system. And it is also about how some individuals and organizations are working to effect change.

And now, dear reader, we invite you to experience nursing from the perspective of these nurses who so graciously share their stories.

# Using This Book

It may sound odd referring to using a book rather than just reading it. However, because of its many resources, you might just dip into this book wherever it seems a good place to start reading. We thought you would appreciate having a way to find these caring resources noted in Part II and where they are discussed in Part I quickly and at-a-glance. You'll find a convient at-a-glance table on the next two pages.

# Caring Resources at a Glance

*Non-Clinical Patient Care*

Advocacy: Nurse advocate, 4, 94

"Art the Cart" (art supplies cart), 98

Caring, intentionality in, 116, 119

Caring, processes of, x, xii, xiii, xiv

Caring, standards for, 84

Humor, use of, 37–38, 46, 59, 97–98, 116, 120–121

Leadership skills, 82–85, 88, 101

Listening, 18, 19, 30, 33, 40, 116, 125

Presence (being present), 33, 49, 89, 116, 119–120

*Non-Clinical Development*

Clinical Ladder of Progression, 94–95

Myers-Briggs Type Indicator,® 84, 112

Nursing Career Interests, 112–114

Self-Caring Audit, 126–127

Self-Care Plan, 127–128

Skill Clusters Inventory, xiv, 108–109

Transferable Skills Card Sort, xiv, 109–112

*Nursing Staff Support/Education*

Administrative rounding, 97

Appreciative Inquiry, 90, 98, 100, 116, 119

Cascade learning, 85

Communication skills, 83–85

Leadership core competencies, 83–86

Preceptor programs, 62, 95

Story sharing, 116–118

Students (new) and caring, 92–93

*Organizational Caring and Enhancement*

Chief Retention Officer, 83

Compassionate Communication, 86

Employment interview process (Engaged Selection), 85

Healing Environment, 81, 86, 89

Nominal Group Technique, 92–93

Physician involvement, 83

Storytelling, 1–2, 68, 85–86, 106–107, 116, 117–118

Suggestion program (Bright Ideas), 85

*Other Healing Modalities*

Allergies Elimination (NAET), 28–29

AMMA Therapy, ®™ 12,

Healing touch, 12, 17, 25, 38, 49, 98

Holistic healing cart, 14

Forgiveness, 116, 122

Foot Reflexology, 12, 13

Integrative imagery, 12–13, 14

Meditation, 116, 122

Music, 14, 86, 89, 116, 126

Prayer, 24, 25, 28, 32, 44, 45, 64, 67, 116, 121

*Nurses Called to Care: Resources*

*Callings* (Levoy), 104

*The Soul's Code* (Hillman), 104

*Hearing From the Heart* (Farrington), 104

*Finding Your Calling* (Finney), 104

Jean Watson, 94, 99, 118, 123, 133

International Association for Human Caring, 123–24

Relationship-Centered Care Network, 124

Nurse Manifest Network, 124

# About the Authors

**Linda S. Henry**. Linda is Principal of Marketing and Communication Strategies, Puyallup, Washington. She has over 18 years of extensive healthcare education, communication, and marketing experience in for-profit and not-for-profit organizations in diverse settings. As a consultant, she works with hospitals, hospital corporations, and medical practices. Her specialties include strategic business planning and enhancing customer satisfaction. She is a published author and an experienced workshop facilitator.

**James D. Henry**. Jim is Principal of Positive Strategies Unlimited, Puyallup, Washington. He has more than 25 years' experience in management training, organizational enhancement, and career development. For 10 years, he was training manager for Texas Utilities (now TXU), a Fortune 500 company. Most recently, he served as a career planning specialist with Washington Mutual Bank. An experienced trainer, Jim facilitates workshops and conference presentations on a variety of topics.

Linda and Jim are co-recipients of the 2001 Ida and Cecil Green Honors Lectureship, Texas Christian University, College of Health and Human Sciences. Together and individually, they facilitate workshops and conferences on such topics as Leading and Retaining Employees, Reclaiming Soul in Health Care, Organizational Caring from the Inside Out, and The Power of the Caring Nurse.

Jim and Linda are authors of two previous books, *The Soul of the Physician: Doctors Speaking About Passion, Resilience and Hope* (AMA Press 2002) and *Reclaiming Soul in Health Care; Practical Strategies for Revitalizing Providers of Care* (AHA Press 1999).

# Part I
## Nurses Stories From the Heart

*Gentle gestures drift from one to another.*
   *listening*
   *gazing*
   *touching*
   *holding*
*Feelings rendered, in, around, and through.*
   *warmth*
  *interest*
*concern*
*caring*
*Shared moments converge. I and you becomes we.*
*Actions offered, regard given, love bestowed,*
  *create a trickle of compassion,*
   *that feeds a river of kindness,*
    *that courses to the sea of humanity,*
    *and in mingling with the vastness,*
     *purifies all.*

—Kathy Sitzman, RN, Assistant Nursing Professor,
Weber State University, Ogden, Utah
and home healthcare nurse
(Printed with permission)

Storytelling is seen [by some nurses] as unsophisticated and unworthy of nursing, especially because nurses have been trying so desperately to gain respect as a scientific discipline, under the assumption that such respect will earn us a greater role in healthcare decision making.

But storytelling is not the shameful little sister of science. Stories can show policymakers and administrators the impact of their decisions and can be part of error analysis. Patients write in journals to find meaning in their illnesses and to promote healing. And a growing number of nurses are writing narratives about their work to better understand what constitutes expert practice and for promotions . . .

What good are our stories if we don't use them to raise important issues in the right venues with the right people? If we reduce what we do to mere numbers, what will we really know about health, illness, and nursing?[1]

Diana J. Mason, PhD, RN, FAAN, AJN Editor-in-Chief
(*American Journal of Nursing*, 2003; printed with permission)

# Midwife at the Exit

## Christine Hall, BA, RN, CHPN
### *Wounded healer who paints her patients*

"I was in my twenties when both of my parents were killed in a car accident," recounts Chris Hall. "I felt a very deep connection with them. Their death was especially untimely because it came at a time when I was transitioning from my parents being guardians and directors of my life to parents as partners. Their loss became a pivotal point in my life where, all of a sudden, I felt very alone, and I was forced to move into a kind of unformed fogginess in order to discover who I truly was as a person."

It was not, however, until she was in her forties that her journey led her into nursing. Although not a typical career path, Chris entered hospice work immediately upon graduating from nursing school. "Hospice management understood that I had passed through this dark night of the soul because of my earlier personal experience with grief," she says, "and allowed me to begin with hospice work."

After a couple of years, Chris decided to broaden her work experience by entering rehabilitation nursing. However, she found it to be too structured and not as satisfying to her heart and soul as was hospice. She explains, "During rehab nursing, I watched a couple of patients die. The doctors approached the patients' families about whether they wanted to continue rehab or move into palliative care. I observed family members not knowing what to do. In earlier times, the physician would take the lead and suggest what would be best for the patient. We don't do that any more, but simply identify the options.

"I watched people make decisions based upon their hope," Chris continues. "I remember one patient's wife making the worst possible decision in the presence of the doctor; I desperately wanted to interrupt because I *knew* what the man's vital signs were, but that would have been inappropriate because I wasn't invited to participate. We pulled the man out of his bed, sat him in a chair, and continued with his rehabilitation. Having had two years hospice experience, I knew it would be a disaster, but I followed the doctor's orders anyway, sticking the man with a needle nine times trying to get a blood sample as his vessels were attempting to close. He was holding weights in his hands when he died. His wife had gone somewhere to take a nap and when she returned, we had to inform her that her husband had died. It was so wrong," she recounts sadly.

As a result of this experience, Chris realized that she wanted no part of such a system and that her place was in hospice where she could truly attend to people who are attempting to cope.

Chris totally agrees with the concept of nurse advocate, an expanded role that is particularly needed today for an aging population with declining health. A nurse advocate on a monthly retainer would be available to serve as a guide and counselor assisting families to navigate through the complex medical system and to make appropriate decisions along the way.

"There is a very strong need for this service," she proclaims. "In fact, one of the things I love to speak about to young nurses coming out of school is becoming a nurse who can help guide people through the maze of health care. It is so fragmented and people become very frightened by it. Often the patient has no idea of where to go next. A nurse advocate who can assess the situation and the recommendations of doctors can advise, 'Well, that's one idea. Now let's look at a few more possibilities.' It allows the patient and his or her family to see the big picture and the totality of their options, including the introduction of nonclinical modalities, such as meditation, guided imagery, or music therapy."

Chris believes strongly in the importance of orchestrating one's end-of-life experiences, making decisions ahead of time about how one wishes to die, including the use of these different adjunct therapies. For example, if you want music therapy, then what kind of music would you prefer if you were unable to communicate your desires to others? Therapeutic touch might be very appropriate for one person but not for another.

| Skill Clusters | Transferable Skills |
|---|---|
| Artistic | Performing |
| Creativity | Dependability |
| Communication | Aesthetic Judgment |
| Learning | Designing/Drawing |
| Self-directing | Synthesizing |
| Compassion | |
| Idea-oriented | |

Considering Chris's skill clusters of *artistic* and *creativity* coupled with transferable skills related to *aesthetic judgment* and *designing/drawing*, it is not surprising that she discovered artistic expression as a vital way of revitalizing and balancing herself. "In the first place, those of us in hospice practice tend to be wounded healers," she asserts. "Studies demonstrate that many hospice nurses gravitate to this profession because we are in the process of healing ourselves. I was not conscious of this initially, but have become much more so as time passes. I find tremendous power and healing in hospice, especially by including and nurturing my artistic interests and talents. It is part of the nature of hospice to be immersed in the wounding cycle because the expected outcome involves losing our patients. Yet, we cannot prevent ourselves from truly loving at least some of them. My use of art works like a soothing salve to some of the troubled areas of my soul.

"I have created an artistic symbol system of painting animals that represent some of my patients," she says with a smile. "These pictures remind me of something I have learned from them that I need to know. For example, one patient taught me how important it is to use our personal creativity because you can control it, much more so than controlling destructive impulses. In this troubled and broken world, most of us are attempting to gain some kind of control over our lives. I captured this lesson in the art form by painting a raccoon. This patient was a creature of the night with dexterous hands, an artist himself. He was 29 years old."

The wife of one of Chris's patients became ill while caring for her husband. "She didn't inform me of her situation until near the end of her husband's life. I referred her to a physician who determined that the woman had stage four abdominal cancer. I asked her why she had not told me about her pain earlier. She said that she did not want any time and resources to be taken away from her husband. Then she said, 'You must understand that I do not choose to outlive my husband by much because he was my best friend.' I told her that was something I really needed to hear. I had become really attached to her and believed for my sake that she needed to live longer. When she told me about her desire to die, I was able to focus upon her needs, not mine."

After the woman's death, Chris painted a picture of a cow that symbolized this woman. She relates, "There is something about the cow I painted that in my mind aligns with the essence of that woman. For me, painting such pictures becomes the way I share my hospice stories and the lessons I have learned from them. It doesn't happen immediately, but takes some time before I realize I must paint and share a patient's story. I go through a murky, gestational period, sometimes for a week or month and other times for years. When ready, the art then emerges from inside my psyche."

Another of her patients was Joe, diagnosed with terminal cancer, who was the son of one of Chris's dear nurse friends, also an artist. Chris was Joe's hospice nurse. She explains, "For Joe, I came up with the image of a horse. His parents constructed a ramp from his bed down five or six steps to the living room, and when we took his wheelchair down the ramp, it sounded like horses walking from a truck ramp to a corral. So, I came up with the idea of Joe as a draft horse."

Chris always viewed her nursing and her artistic tendencies as polar opposites. However, while forming a relationship with three nursing companions who are also artistically inclined, the idea of bringing artistic forms to nursing began to swirl together. The group now often speaks to nurses about renewing their nursing passion through art. The idea of picturing Joe as a draft horse materialized as one of her early drawings. One member of the foursome is ICU nurse Lisa Wayman, Joe's mother; her story comes next.

Susan Conde, retired hospice nurse, poet, and author, is also part of the group. Her poem *Midwives at the Exit* describes Chris well.

> Hospice nurses . . .
> midwives at the exit
> ushering souls,
> eager or reluctant,
> forward
> as footlights fade.
> Never hastening,
> always encouraging,
> one last look around . . .
> the errant glove,
> the forgotten hat,
> anything left or neglected.
>
> Angels of the inevitable . . .
> well aware
> a gentle passing
> from darkened corridor
> to haloed exit
> depends so much
> on so little . . .
> a single gesture,
> a simple declaration,
> or just
> goodbye.
>
> —Reprinted with permission

# JOE'S MOM—A STORY OF TRANSFORMATION

Lisa M. Wayman, MSN, RN

*ICU nurse: A mother's pain, a professional's passsion*

As a Navy brat, Lisa Wayman moved frequently in her early years, eventually settling in upstate New York. She entered nursing later in life, somewhat reluctantly. "I graduated from nursing school when I was 30," she says. "I know nurses who believe they are called to the profession, but back then, I was not one of them. I graduated from college as a teacher, but shortly thereafter, I got married, had babies, and decided I did not want to take care of children both day and night. So, I reluctantly entered nursing school knowing that I would be very good at it clinically."

Upon graduation, Lisa went immediately into critical care. "I loved it," she exclaims. "You had to use your head all of the time, and you had so much high-tech equipment to tinker with. I could play with ventilators, IV pumps, and all the other paraphernalia found there. For about the first year, it was really fun. Unfortunately, I can't remember any of my patients or their stories during that period because all I concentrated on were the machines. Emotionally, I put up a wall between myself and my patients."

One of Lisa's nursing professors was Lea Gaydos, who was named national holistic nurse of the year in 1998. "She lectured on the importance of caring. I remember actually raising my hand during the class, asking her to please get to the point. I believed nursing was no more than a 'doing for' profession and that patients didn't need caring for in any other manner."

After a year into her career, Lisa began to dread going to work. It became very painful because the wall she had created isolated her from others. She was a professional and determined not to get involved in people's emotional traumas. Then she began experiencing nightmares and losing sleep at night. She tells us, "Horrible things were happening around me at work; people were critically ill and dying, but I could not cry or express any emotion. I thought about leaving nursing, so in desperation I went back to my nursing professor, Lea, for some advice. She reminded me again that nursing is not just about clinical work and technology, but also about caring. She said the nurse is the tool of nursing. But how could I be a tool? I felt totally empty with nothing to give."

One thing Lisa did do was engage in some self-care. She began to exercise and meditate. She took more time with her family and went to a counselor. "Eventually, I began to see some of my patients as real people," she gently recalls. "Many of my patients ended up in ICU because of their bad habits, but I became less judgmental of them. I began to see how we are all connected and there but for the grace of God go I. It was my job to care and not to try to figure out who deserved it. I was on the way, taking some baby steps toward becoming a caring nurse."

However, just as Lisa began making these small strides, the roof suddenly caved in on her. Her son, Joe, having just turned 11 years old, was diagnosed with a brain stem tumor. She describes entering an incredibly difficult journey through the dark night of the soul. "The treatment for this kind of cancer is simply ugly, with chemo, radiation, and, worst of all, the use of steroids," she relates tearfully. "Because of the steroids, Joe's weight went from 85 pounds to 185 pounds. Within 18 months, he passed away."

As difficult as that period in her life was, Lisa believes that she learned a great deal from the experience. Joe's life and death became a gift to both Lisa and her patients because it helped her move through a transformation process from being a cold, uncaring clinician to becoming a much more human person of compassion. She states, "It was a journey through the dark night of the soul that I would not like to repeat, but it caused my growth to speed up. With Joe, I initially thought that the only good outcome would be his return to health. But I learned to let go and not try to control the outcome of an event. That was very difficult because I am the oldest child of the family, and I always wanted to be in charge. As an ICU nurse, I knew what needed to be done and I did it. But I simply could do nothing to make my son live. So, I have learned to live in the present.

"Today when I live in the present moment with my patients, I am much better able to be a channel for healing even though many of them will not be cured. My job is not to try to fix them, but to help people heal in any way appropriate. Sometimes that means healing their bodies; I still do all of the clinical things competently. But, it could mean helping to heal relationships, especially with family members. Other times it involves healing the spirit, which can be profoundly difficult."

By spirit, Lisa believes that there exists a divine element in everything. After death, that part of us which is divine continues in some fashion. She believes that we are here on earth to learn lessons and that we may return to earth or to some other dimension of existence to continue learning. "When he was dying, Joe would ask me what happens after death," she tells us. "I told him that I don't know what happens, but that I trusted he would be okay. That's what faith is: stepping off into the dark and trusting that you will be caught. By the time Joe was about to die, he was ready because his body was not serving him.

"The other thing I learned from Joe was not to take myself quite so seriously and to laugh a lot more. When he first started chemotherapy, he lost all of his hair and it was Halloween. He decided to dress up as his father, who has no hair. But Dad had a beard, so we bought Joe a fake beard and he dressed like his computer programmer father. I learned from this and other experiences with him that if you have to be in control, you remain serious all of the time. But if you can let go of that, even for a short period of time, then you can lighten up and have some fun."

Continuing, Lisa says, "Of course, I never laugh directly at my patients. But I sometimes laugh out loud at myself, make jokes about the equipment making dumb sounds, or name the IV pole. People in ICU are scared, and laughter can make them feel more comfortable."

Lightening up and letting go also allowed Lisa to recover her artistic skills. During Joe's illness she began to work primarily with oils. It was one way to display and express her emotions, both grief and joy. Her art also helped her return to work in ICU even as Joe's illness progressed. She never received formal art training, and it was never about hanging a piece of art on a gallery wall, she explains. Rather, it was about feeding the soul.

As a result of her journey leading up to Joe's death, Lisa became more and more disenchanted with the intensive care environment. Too much focus was placed upon physical issues, she realized. "We ask the *how* questions—what else can be done for the patient, but not the *why* questions—why should we do this procedure in light of the reality that death will probably come in the near future."

So she returned to her mentor, Lea, for guidance, who suggested that she return to school and begin working on a master's degree in holistic nursing. "I began with a course called Dynamics of Unity, a highly interactive class on consciousness and interconnectedness of all things. Holistic theory is often best expressed in art forms and other experiential modalities, so I was able to use even more of my *artistic* and *aesthetic judgment* and skills."

| Skill Clusters | Transferable Skills |
| --- | --- |
| Connectivity | Negotiating |
| Idea-oriented | Explaining |
| Leadership | Synthesizing |
| Learning | Using Experience |
| Communication | Aesthetic Judgment |
| Flexibility | |

As a result of her transformational journey, not surprisingly *connectivity* surfaces as one of Lisa's key skill clusters. "Often," she informs us, "I walk into a patient's room and I feel this strong connection with her or him, even though the individual may be asleep or unconscious. We are all different facets of that one spirit that I mentioned earlier."

Today, Lisa continues working in ICU but is able to use her *leadership, communication,* and life *experience* skills in a much different manner. "I work from a holistic paradigm," she explains. "Actually, now I have a reputation of and specialty for taking care of dying patients. Some staff members laughingly call me the death nurse, but I don't cause people to die. I simply precede the angel of death. I work with patients and families who have very difficult decisions to make. I also work under a research grant that allows me to visit people in their homes, providing some symptom management and discussing end-of-life issues."

At present, Lisa maintains her clinical competence but has transitioned to the point of helping people to die in comfort, peace, and fulfillment. In fact, her master's thesis is on self-transcendence through suffering. It is not about people getting stuck in the dark night of the soul, but about people who have come out of it into the light. "It's like an earthquake, having a huge shift in one's identity and orientation," she notes.

Lisa also teaches a class for student nurses. "I share my story and demand that they care. I tell them that you can nurse people without caring but it will tear you apart, so you may as well cry when it's a sad situation and laugh when it's happy. Yes, we have to maintain some boundaries, but they must be flexible and not prevent us from being human, becoming involved and connected to the patient."

# Dancing with the Atoms in the Universe

## Deborah McElligott, RN, ANP, HNP
### *Holistic nurse practitioner: Visionary with a healing plan*

"I want to dance with the atoms in the universe, resonate with God's power of love, all healing, all giving, showering down upon me daily, as long as my umbrella isn't up,©" says acute-care nurse practitioner Debbie McElligott, describing her personal philosophy.

During two-and-a-half years of holistic nurse training, Debbie engaged in a long period of stress reduction and self-assessment. "At one point," she reports, "we had to develop a statement of life's purpose, something that would provide direction for the rest of our lives. I want to feel and share the love, remembering that it is here and available so long as I am not walking around protecting myself, with my umbrella always up.

"Of course," she adds, "sometimes you need the umbrella. We need to protect ourselves, not from God's love, but from some of the destructive forces of the universe. But if we continually use this metaphorical umbrella as a shield, we find ourselves in a very sad state of affairs, unable to partake of the joy and fruits of creation and of our community with it."

In retrospect, Debbie cannot remember ever wanting to be a nurse. "I know it's strange," she recounts, "but I never really wanted to put a bandage on a person. My mother always wanted to be a nurse, but chose to care for her family instead. I wanted to teach English, but didn't want to attend college for four years, so as a matter of practicality, I decided to attend a three-year nursing program. There weren't that many choices for women back in the 1960s, and nursing represented something you could do part-time if you wanted to raise a family. Two weeks before starting school, my father took me to the city to meet Mrs. Kirkwood, an elderly nursing leader who insisted that I attend a four-year program. So I attended Hunter-Bellevue College."

Debbie didn't particularly enjoy the sciences but loved being with people. "I came from a very caring, loving family," she underscores. "Caring became my joy and passion in life."

Most of Debbie's 30-plus-year nursing career has been spent in the acute cardiac care of open-heart surgery patients within her home state of New York. Responding to the technical demands of this work, Debbie advanced her clinical skills by becoming a nurse practitioner. "We managed the patients before and after surgery, a very difficult role because of the many serious responsibilities associated with their care, including admitting and discharging them, and writing orders and prescriptions. There were long hours and a fear of making mistakes or overlooking a potential problem. It was frustrating work, and it resulted in almost a total ignoring of one's own care. Everything was fast paced with little time available for breaks. You became regimented, and as the day wore on, it became a greater struggle to truly care for a patient beyond his or her clinical needs. Your soul seems to be diminished after working so hard for four or five days in a row."

However, a significant turn of events has occurred in Debbie's life/work journey over the past five years during which time she has entered a holistic nursing program. Having learned therapeutic touch in the 1980s, she found the environment was not conducive to implementing this therapy. Finding such tunnel-vision atmosphere softening in the 1990s, she completed course work in AMMA Therapy®™, Foot Reflexology, and Integrative Imagery, with a view toward more holistic nursing.

AMMA Therapy®™ is a comprehensive healing art that combines Oriental medical principles based on the balance and flow of energy, with a Western approach of assessing organ dysfunction. Like acupuncture, it focuses on the balance and movement of energy within the body. Whereas the acupuncturist inserts needles into the energy pathways to stimulate and move the energy, the AMMA therapist relies primarily on the sensitivity and strength of the hands to manipulate the life energy.

Foot Reflexology is a "pressure therapy" and involves applying focused pressure and massage to certain known "reflex" points located on the foot, which correspond to certain other areas in the body. Some of the recognized benefits from receiving a reflexology treatment include increased circulation, relaxation, and tension release.

Working in a conservative East Coast hospital, Debbie astutely knew it would be better to implement alternative therapies slowly. She decided to begin with imagery. "I introduced audio tapes that were being used nationwide. We conducted a research study and, although the results were statistically insignificant, we were able to offer the tapes to all of our patients about 18 months later from donated funds."

Then Debbie and a team of nursing investigators introduced AMMA Therapy®™ to 30 nurses and studied its impact. "We had both a study group and control group. We asked the people in the study group to describe their experiences with the treatment and its impact upon their nursing efforts," she states, "and they reported increased body/mind connections. Some felt more energized and at peace. At first, even the people in the control group spoke initially about having pleasant experiences, but they failed to follow through with all the treatments. The study received recognition from the hospital, and it was presented at both national and international conferences."

Today, Debbie's professed love continues to be in the areas of holistic nursing involving therapeutic patient care and education. "I love to write my own PowerPoint presentations to address learning and therapeutic issues," she exclaims. "I conduct workshops on Integrative Imagery and do a series on holistic healing looking at body, mind, and spirit. Healing is an integrative process in which people need to take responsibility for their health and develop a healing plan with the help of their health-care practitioners. It involves more than taking pills."

Expanding on foot reflexology, Debbie explains, "The foot serves as a map to the body. Reflexes on the foot mirror the whole body; for example, the reflexes relating to the head are on the toes. It serves as another way of assessing patients, determining what is going on, and healing. People may resonate with different types of modalities, so the clue is to know what works for you and make it part of your health plan. Everyone has their own path to healing."

Debbie's personal path to healing and wholeness includes integrating spiritual and religious orientations. "I don't believe that you can separate them. I am a Eucharistic minister in the Roman Catholic Church. I love my religion, and the older I become, the more I find it to be a real source of comfort. I notice that many people growing up in the 1950s and 1960s speak of fearing God, but I always envisioned a God who cares and nurtures."

As with other nurses we interviewed, Debbie would never impose her beliefs upon another person, but she does envision her faith, nursing, and life in general as flowing together in a very positive nurturing way. This is why, for a period of time during a low point in her nursing career, she was attracted to Mary Kay Cosmetics. Mary Kay's philosophy revolved around the Golden Rule, to "do unto others as you would have them do unto you."

Debbie tells us, "At the monthly meetings you could only share good stories and give positive feedback. Mary Kay's priorities were faith first, family second, and career third. You weren't expected to put your career ahead of your husband and children. At one point I thought about quitting nursing and going full time with Mary Kay. This was the kind of energy I wanted to be part of. I became so involved that I had to choose one or the other, and my true passion was with holistic nursing. My priorities became faith, family, and nursing. I strongly feel that the philosophy, priorities, and support system of Mary Kay nourished me and are qualities that I want to bring to nursing through the role of the holistic nurse practitioner."

| Skill Clusters | Transferable Skills |
|---|---|
| Visionary | Drive/Tenacity |
| Conviction | Initiating |
| Self-direction | Planning |
| Learning | Emotional Control |
| Achievement | Synthesizing |
| Leadership | |
| Artistic | |

It is not surprising that Debbie's key skill clusters include *conviction* and being a *visionary*. However, she uses these skills inclusively and not exclusively. She enjoys utilizing her *drive* and *leadership* skills to *synthesize*, bringing together the various healing traditions and modalities. She views it as the purpose of holistic nursing and integrative medicine; it's not East versus West, but a combination of both.

Debbie developed a "holistic healing cart" in her cardiac unit that volunteers take to patients. First made available to the nursing staff as a way of educating them about various caring and healing modalities, it also serves as a resource for staff self-care. "The cart is stocked with relaxation items, guided imagery and humor audiotapes, books on a variety of healing modalities, as well as books with pretty pictures and pencil and paper for people to draw or doodle or whatever they wish," she explains. "Of course it has Bibles, books, and materials on prayer and spirituality, anything that serves to inspire people and focus upon healing the body, mind, and spirit. We have a committee of interested people, including chaplains, social workers, and patient educators, who provide input for which items to include."

Debbie maintains that there is an endless number of resources and tools available to help people heal. "Even if patients don't take advantage of them while in the hospital, we encourage them to return for outpatient classes, and perhaps then they become more open to existing resources.

"You never know what will touch someone. I had an older patient once who didn't find anything of interest on the cart. But, then I found him listening to "Amazing Grace" with a Latino beat!" she laughs. "We have to be careful that we don't stereotype people and assume to know what will interest and reach them. So, we try to offer a wide variety of things.

"I am excited about what I am doing at this stage of my life. I have the opportunity to listen to patients in a job I love," she says enthusiastically. "And I am looking forward to introducing and integrating holistic healing within a hospital setting, though I know realistically that it must be done over time and with care. I also know how important it is for me to take care of myself and to balance my personal, family, and professional lives."

# TENACITY WITH A SMILE
## Steven H. Brant, BSN, RN, PHN
### *Navy nurse: Committed optimist*

People sometimes describe Lieutenant Steve Brant, naval officer and nurse, as a person who faces life's problems with a smile on his face. An optimist who thrives upon meeting challenges, he searches for solutions, not accepting "no" for an answer in the midst of adversity. Once, he nursed a Native American Indian who was about to die. "The man was afraid to die in the hospital because, with air conditioning, you can't open the windows," Steve recounts. "The man believed that if he did not die with open windows letting in the outside air, his spirit would not ascend to the afterlife. So, as he gasped for his last few breaths, we pushed his bed at a rather high rate of speed down the hallway and through an open door to the outside. He died in peace, knowing that his spirit would be released."

Steve's determination became severely challenged in February 1991 when his 7-year-old son became ill with leukemia. On the Sunday before Steve was scheduled to leave for Saudi Arabia and Desert Storm, the pastor made an announcement during the worship service for him and his wife to go to the education wing and to care for their son. "It was embarrassing to have hundreds of people staring at us as we went down the aisle," he recalls. "Our son's teacher told us that he had taught for 20 years and never before summoned parents from a church service, but Greg was vomiting and something told him to send for us. The next day we took him to the doctor for tests. I looked at one of the x-rays and it appeared as though someone had placed a shoebox over my son's heart. He actually had two different cancers, a tumor on the thymus gland, which is why we could not see his heart, as well as t-cell leukemia."

Steve was excused from going overseas, and his son began chemotherapy treatment weekly for three years. Breaking down with emotion, he relates, "Greg had to go to the operating room once a month for a spinal tap to determine the presence of cancer. One day as we got on the elevator, he pushed the button for the pediatric floor as opposed to the operating room floor. When we informed him that we were stopping at the wrong level, he said, 'I know, Dad, but I want to stop here to get my angel.'"

Continuing tearfully, Steve states, "Whether or not you believe in guardian angels, I am thoroughly convinced that the worldwide prayer chain we had in place during this period made a difference. Even some of my buddies in Saudi Arabia participated in it.

"Greg had a Hickman catheter for three years that I took care of. Amazingly, he never had an infection even though he lived a normal life that included swimming and surfing at the beach. Today he is fine—just turned 20 years old, is 6 feet 4 inches tall, and weighs 240 pounds. He plays goalie for an amateur hockey league and attends college, working toward a degree in graphic design," Steve says proudly.

Steve's earliest recollection of wanting to enter health care evolved from his feeling of helplessness as a child when someone was hurt or ill. He wanted to do more than simply console them. Growing up on a ranch in Southern Oregon and tending to animals further reinforced this desire. After high school, he worked for a logging company to supplement his ranch income. He was eventually selected as their safety director, which required him to receive training as an Emergency Medical Technician (EMT). Finally, after working with the local ambulance service, he knew he wanted to become a nurse and joined the Navy in order to attain his education goals.

Choosing the Navy as opposed to another branch of the service has historical precedent. "It's really an interesting story," he laughs. "My great-grandfather skippered a Swedish merchant ship. While sailing in 1862, he rescued some people on a sinking ship, one of whom was the king of a small European country. In gratitude, the king commissioned a picture to be painted of my great-grandfather's ship and also gave him a telescope. Our family tradition is that the first child of each generation who goes to sea becomes the custodian of these treasures. So," he grins, "I felt a call to carry on this tradition and joined the navy, though I have yet to be assigned to sea duty! I am still seeking at least a short-term assignment, because if I fail, supposedly the picture and telescope are to be sent to a maritime museum in Gothenberg Sweden."

| Skill Clusters | Transferable Skills |
|---|---|
| Technical Competence | Rapid Reaction |
| Leadership | Using Experience |
| Accountability | Responding to Emergencies |
| Flexibility | Advising |
| Entrepreneurship | Responding to Pressure |
| Creativity | |
| Idea-oriented | |

From early childhood to the present, Steve's skills provide a foundation for his professional passion. Not surprisingly, his *technical competence*, *flexibility*, *rapid reaction* and *responding to pressure* abilities represent a perfect fit for emergency medicine. He continues using his *leadership* and *creativity* talents as a hands-on clinical administrator at a naval hospital in Oak Harbor, Washington. Steve reports, "I also use these skills as the coordinator of the Sexual Assault Nurse Examiner Team on the base. We must respond rapidly to three or four events each month. That may seem like a lot of assault situations, but it is a large facility, and the rate of occurrences mirrors that of the public in general."

Steve reminds us that in the Navy people live by honor, courage, and commitment. "My primary job involves teaching hospital corpsman how to take care of patients, so if and when they go to sea or with the marines, during peacetime or war, they can care for sailors and marines. Corpsman training allows them to function like a combined EMT and nurse. As a person new to the Navy 20 years ago, that is how I was trained, and now it's my turn to do that for those who work for me."

Along with several other nurses we interviewed, Steve practices therapeutic touch. "At the time I became interested in it, I was a relatively new nurse in the Navy," he relates. "By laying hands on a patient, I can help move the energy fields for better healing. In fact, once the methodology is learned, you can practice therapeutic touch on yourself. It serves as an excellent way of relieving stress, and sometimes I use it to fall asleep more rapidly."

As a male nurse, Steve admits to feeling stereotyped to some degree, but believes stereotyping is currently receding, especially in the military. "In general," he claims, "men represent 6% of the nursing population, whereas in the armed services, that figure is somewhere about 33%. The number of corpsmen and medics who enter the profession impacts that figure."

He reminds us that contrary to popular perception, historically, until the last few centuries, it was mostly men in the medical and nursing professions who took care of the ill. From the time of the earliest settlers in the United States and especially during times of war, men filled nursing positions. It wasn't until 1873 that a woman was identified as the first "trained nurse" in this country.

Again, not surprisingly, another one of Steve's key skill clusters entails *technical competence*. "I love to read," he informs us. "When I read medical literature, I like to read about family practice, internal medicine, and critical care. I enjoy reading material written for physicians because it goes into greater depth than that written for nurses. When I retire from the Navy, my intention is to become a nurse practitioner, probably in urgent care.

"Apart from health care, I read a wide variety of books, most of which are related to the western way of life, such as Zane Gray, Samuel Clemens (Mark Twain), and Will Rogers. Not many people realize it because of stereotyping seen in the movies, but American cowboys and ranchers were people with deep conviction and morality. Like them, I was raised on a ranch and taught by my grandparents and parents to be a very hardworking person."

> *Cowboy's Ten Commandments*
>
> 1. Just 1 God.
> 2. Honor yer Ma & Pa.
> 3. No tellin' tales or gossipin'
> 4. Git yourself to Sunday Meetin'.
> 5. Put nothin' before God.
> 6. No foolin' round with another fella's gal.
> 7. No killin'.
> 8. Watch yer mouth.
> 9. Don't take what ain't yers.
> 10. Don't be hankerin' fer yer buddy's stuff
>
> *Guess cowboys just kinda tell it like it is!*

Steve also reads the Bible every day and remains active in his Christian faith, although he honors other people's orientations and does not impose his belief system upon them. He views soul and spirit as being so closely connected that they are difficult to separate. He affirms, "Soul is that part of me that anchors my strong desire and drive to do what is right. I have the capacity to know when something is wrong and to know when to get others involved to fix the problem."

Because of his tenacious attitude, Steve doesn't believe that the current healthcare environment of staffing shortages, managed care, fiscal constraints, and the like prevents nurses from being caring individuals. "I just don't believe it," he states emphatically. "People who want to bemoan the fact that they are too busy or overtaxed to care need to step back and examine themselves. What motivated them to enter the profession in the first place? Was it the money or perhaps a staffing plan that enabled them to work three days per week? Nurses dedicated to the profession will always find time to care for patients, physically and otherwise. Often it depends upon their time management skills, which are critical in this profession. Demonstrating that you care sometimes only requires five minutes of intense listening. You can determine a patient's frustration fairly quickly; spending a few minutes with them makes all the difference.

"With respect to nursing shortages, I believe we have caused the problem ourselves. When it was decided that, by the 1980s the BSN would be the entry level into the profession, hospital-based diploma programs were forced out of business and little was done to replace them. At the same time, it became very difficult to enter a degree program, so the profession limited itself and caused the shortage problem."

In the midst of health care's accelerating change, Steve still remains optimistic about the future of health care. He says, "We nurses are gaining more autonomy even though the insurance companies are pressuring all healthcare professionals about how to practice medicine. But, at some point, we need to take more of a stand and do what is right for the patient.

"Being a caring nurse is about intensely focusing one's attention and energy upon the patient and the family, in spite of frustrating external pressures," Steve affirms. "Sometimes patients feel lost in attempting to navigate through the system. As nurses, we attempt to serve as their advocates, to find out what is needed, and respond accordingly, even if it is just by providing a listening ear."

# GIVING SMALL GIFTS

### Janet E. Hersh, RN, CNICU, CCRN
*ICU nurse: Empathy and imagination*

"It's amazing how the little things you do really make a difference," states Janet Hersh. "You may not realize it at the time, but they impact others." She relates the story of a woman with cancer who was about to undergo surgery. No family members or friends were with her just before surgery when patients are most fearful. She asked Janet if she would be there when she awoke after surgery. "I only knew her for about 12 hours, but I must have connected meaningfully with her in some small way," she says tearfully. Retelling the story rekindled the emotion of the moment and she confesses, "I told my daughter earlier that I wasn't going to cry during this interview, but she said, 'Mom, you always cry.'"

The giving of small gifts epitomizes caring, Janet believes. "For me, caring involves intuitively approaching people, understanding them, and attempting to meet their needs by giving of oneself. A caring person often goes the extra mile, doing special little things frequently beyond what is expected. You don't have to expend a great amount of energy; often it simply involves listening and often the physical contact that communicates an emotional bonding. Many of the nurses I work with are very caring people who do more than the task at hand, like giving a back rub when it's not required."

Gift giving goes both ways, she avows. "The hospital impacts my life in many positive ways," Janet affirms. "I'm not thinking of anything dramatic, but of many small gifts of giving. One nun, Sister Stella Maris, a very interesting woman who was truly a patient and a staff advocate, said and did little things that made nurses feel special. She had hypertension, always wanting me to take her blood pressure because she said I was gentle and didn't hurt her arm by pumping the pressure too high. Also, Father Cummings, a hospital chaplain, would visit with all the nurses and hospital staff as well as patients. In fact, he became like a father to all of us, helping us to feel like a family. We celebrated his birthday each year by taking a group from the hospital to the Atlanta Braves game. He was such a big sports fan, and he loved spending time with his St. Joseph family. You weren't just a nurse working in a unit, but part of a family who cared for one another in a vibrant sense of mission."

Janet has been on the staff of St. Joseph's Hospital in Atlanta for 25 years, a remarkable testimony to the hospital's retention rate. Many of Janet's best friends also enjoy a long tenure there. "Our unit is a very unique environment because we know each other so well," she reports. "It creates a deep sense of security to be able to walk into a unit and see familiar faces. We are there together, comrades who support and really care about each other. For example, a few weeks ago a nurse in our unit cared for a young patient who died unexpectedly. It was a very emotional situation for the family as well as the hospital staff. It upset her rather deeply. It was evident that a cup of coffee after work was necessary so we could support each other by listening, caring, crying, reviewing, and validating exactly what it is that we do and why our role is so important."

Janet's grandmother indirectly influenced her decision to enter nursing. "My grandmother seemed to be the caregiver of the family, and whenever someone became ill, she could administer a whole host of remedies," Janet remembers. Recalling a Halloween nurse's costume, she laughs, "The uniform was never put away after Halloween. Whenever someone in the family became ill, I would run to put it on and pretend to be the nurse."

Janet specialized in critical care at a time when many medical advances were taking place. She liked the excitement, the nursing intensity, and delighted in the great amount of learning that took place, all factors that kept her in the critical care arena as a lifelong career. "You find yourself positioned to truly make a difference with patients and family because you relate to people often in the worst circumstances. This is true not only medically, but emotionally, broadening the scope of caring," she relates.

Janet's personal growth reflects a personal tragedy. "I gave birth to a set of premature twins. Our son died at the age of 11 months [today, the twin daughter is 16 years old]. He became very ill, and we eventually faced decisions about prolonging his care and his life. Shortly after I returned to work following his death, I met a woman facing a similar decision about her critically ill husband. I knew the surgeon very well, and he was about to take the family into the waiting room to explain the situation and possible alternatives. The doctor wanted me to join him in talking with the wife, but I objected because the recent situation with my son was still too painful. However, he grabbed me by the arm and insisted that I join him and the family. Anxiously, I entered the waiting room. After hearing about the possibility of removing her husband from the ventilator, she broke down, turned to me, and said, 'You can't imagine how I feel.' Understanding her dilemma and somewhat teary-eyed, I looked her straight in the eye and replied, 'Oh yes I can,'" Janet recounts. "So, my own life experiences make it a little easier to understand what others may be going through."

Janet's experience is a vivid example of empathy, a word derived from two root words: *Em,* meaning "inside," and *pathos,* meaning "feelings." Empathy is that human ability to share inside feelings with others as if we are inside that person's skin. It involves imagining and feeling the pain, the pleasure, the conflicts, and an entire range of very complex feelings. So the statement "I understand" is technically not correct unless we have actually had a similar experience or have used our imagination to feel what it must be like. The French call empathy "imagination sympathique." Whether experienced firsthand or through genuine imagination, empathy is one of the higher forms of caring.

To some degree, empathy can be learned by asking people, "How would you feel if you were in the place of _____?" Asking such a question on a regular basis builds human sensitivity, especially needed in the field of health care, to counterbalance impersonal and technocratic environments.

Janet's modesty about how she touches others' lives undoubtedly was one of the factors leading to her being honored in 2000 as the second recipient of the Ernest W. Franklin III Award for Nursing Excellence. The Franklin Award honorees are chosen to represent the mission of Saint Joseph's nursing staff and their dedication to excellence and compassion in the care of their patients.

Working a flexible schedule allows plenty of family time and time to attend church on Sunday mornings. "On the other hand," she emphasizes, "you must dedicate yourself to go home and sleep! Sleep derivation can be a significant problem for nurses. I may sound like a recruiter, but on the other hand, scheduling flexibility serves as quite an advantage for nurses." Since self-care is an important ingredient to caring for others, she finds time within her schedule to play tennis and other sports.

| Skill Clusters | Transferable Skills |
|---|---|
| Conviction | Emotional Control |
| Compassiion | Verifying |
| Service/Dedication | Dependability |
| Achievement-oriented | Serving |
| Technical Competence | Responding to Emergencies |
| Creativity | |
| Idea-oriented | |

One of Janet's key satisfying skill clusters revolves around *conviction*. She enjoys living in harmony with personal values and operating at high levels of integrity. At times, she cares for patients who have life-threatening illnesses. Conviction directly relates to helping others maintain belief, allowing them to make their own decisions relative to care. It means allowing families to ventilate and support their family member when faced with end-of-life issues.

One would hope that all nurses, especially those working in critical care, would identify *dependability* as a high-level skill. Janet views it in terms of being conscientious, attentive, intuitive, and a multifaceted resource. "I'm fairly brutal when it comes to knowing what you are doing, why you are doing it, and if you don't know, ask," she insists firmly. "It comes with experience. After 25 years on the job, people turn to you because you've covered the territory for a long time. Dependability also means being available to your manager and offering to work extra time when it is required."

*Compassionate* people are sometimes rather soft-spoken, and this characteristic certainly applies to Janet. Compassion not only implies being a good listener, but also means staying fairly calm in the face of difficulty and emergencies. Janet's gentle calmness is especially effective when approaching family members following the death of a loved one. Compassionate responses are especially important with cardiac patients, because one minute they may be enjoying a meal at a restaurant or playing golf and the next minute they suffer a heart attack. In a very frightening way, having a heart attack can suddenly turn someone's life upside down. "So, compassion is not just a matter of taking someone's blood pressure or giving them a pill; it's really *being with* them," she notes.

Janet always attempts to find new and better solutions to situations and problems, including enhanced ways to provide a service. It relates to her skill clusters of being *idea-oriented*. She is an excellent catalyst for positive change. It also pertains to her orientation toward *creativity*, and for her, it means considering and creating new ideas and/or approaches to problems, especially those related to people.

Janet's many talents remind us of the Gallup Corporation's research on what makes for superior customer (and patient) satisfaction. In their book *First, Break All the Rules* (1999)[2], Marcus Buckingham and Curt Coffman recommend that organizations turn their customers into "advocates." Because of the service they have received, these people become intensely loyal and are the organization's largest unpaid public relations workforce.

"I cannot think of any other profession, except perhaps teaching, where you have such an opportunity to impact people's lives, often in crisis situations," she states emphatically. "I am glad to be a little part of that."

# EMPOWERING PRESENCE OF HEART
## Diane M. Newman, BSN, RN
*Cardiac nurse: Work as a kind of love*

The gold heart-shaped pendant that Diane Newman wears along with a simple cross testifies to her life and work purpose, the source of her energy, and her passion for nursing. It seems no accident that she currently cares for cardiac patients at Baylor Hospital in Dallas, Texas. Diane believes that the heart is much more than an organ; it serves as a metaphor for our emotional and spiritual core as well.

Diane spent her early childhood in Nogales, Arizona. "My parents were deeply connected to the Roman Catholic tradition and faith," she says. "They had a profound love of God, and I was a witness to a loving heart that sprang from their convictions. This was especially true when my younger brother, Edward, Jr., was born with a physical deformity. The attending physician counseled that he be placed in an institution and said that he probably would not live beyond seven years of age. My parents disagreed, believing that God had given them this child for a purpose, and they would take care of him. My father believed that Edward was a gift—a learning experience and a challenge. As such, my father and mother shaped my beliefs and values, providing a foundation for my decision to become a nurse. And, in fact, Edward lived to the age of 35."

She continues, "As an adult, I once read an article that the siblings of handicapped children grow up either becoming embittered or developing the same desire to reach out and help others. My situation was the latter. I was really blessed by my parents' love for both of us."

Diane's father also impressed upon her the belief that we are the body of Christ, his representatives on earth. She affirms, "We are here for a purpose, to be here for other people. Another word for it is *presence*. That is what we are all about, being present in someone else's life. At the end of my life, I hope people will say that I was present for them and stood in their imaginary choir as a cheerleader. I would also like them to state that I loved a challenge. Tell me that it can't be done and I will do my best to get it done. It's become my challenge to both my friends and patients, my motto, saying to them, 'You can do it!'"

By the age of 14, Diane knew she wanted a nursing career. After graduating from the University of Arizona College of Nursing, she first worked in pediatrics and then public health.

Diane's long-standing interest in the heart motivated her move to cardiology. "My family has a history of heart problems," she reports. "My Dad has had a heart attack and we've had 10 uncles who died from them. In addition," she adds with a smile, "I love to learn, and there was a lot of work being done in cardiology around 1992.

"I have always desired 'to operate from my heart' with the people I come in contact with. I attempt to make direct eye contact with individuals when I'm speaking with them, because looking into someone's eyes is like penetrating the soul; eyes are the gateway to the heart and soul and convey so much information about the person."

| *Skill Clusters* | *Transferable Skills* |
|---|---|
| Conviction | Drive/Tenacity |
| Compassion | Aesthetic Judgment |
| Communication | Potential Problem-solving |
| Relating | Motor Coordination |
| Accountability | Understanding/Tact |
| Learning | |
| Naturist | |

*Relating* to others and *compassion* serve as two of Diane's key skill clusters. Fortunately, with a few exceptions, over the years she learned how to use these talents without becoming overly involved to the point of burnout. She reports, "When I started my career in pediatric nursing, my first patient was a little boy who had stepped on a hot electrical wire after a storm. The charge entered his foot and exited from the back of his head. He remained on life support for three months. When it became obvious that he was not going to live, his parents asked the pediatrician to remove their son from life support, but he refused. Two other nurses and I approached the physician to reinforce the parents' request. After breaking down in tears, the doctor finally agreed, and we joined him in grieving.

"I went home that evening having developed a severe pain in the back of my head. After seeing a doctor who prescribed Valium®, I began questioning myself. I didn't need the Valium; I was simply grieving the loss of this boy. So I leaned into the pain and eventually it went away. In any case, this is what keeps me tied to nursing. It is the opportunity to exchange feelings and thoughts at a very deep level."

For Diane, being a caring, compassionate nurse means doing things such as praying with a patient when appropriate. With some sadness, she says, "In earlier times we were to be able to do that, but then it became frowned upon. Fortunately, this is beginning to change, and today the hospital is more accepting. So many physicians—and nurses—in cardiology and neurology see so much suffering that they tend to put up a shield. It can be very frustrating for a cardiac nurse to witness a doctor display an objective, unfeeling, all-business attitude. However, I am seeing a return to the softer, compassionate side of caring, the praying, the laying on of hands, and the like."

Diane's key skill of *aesthetic judgment* means seeing beauty in everything. She attempts to see beyond the surface condition or presenting issue, asking, "What is beautiful and noteworthy about this person?" Diane credits her mother, whose advice counseled, "Look to see what is good about a person."

Diane identifies *naturist* as a key skill cluster and *motor coordination* as a satisfying, specific ability, which is one of the main ways she takes care of herself. She loves to walk, especially in the early morning or at night, becoming one with surroundings and marveling in gratitude for the gifts that God has given us. She walks about 10 miles every weekend. "My dad was an athlete in college, and I learned from him how physical exercise is a great way to reduce stress." She enjoys outside activities requiring motor coordination, a skill she learned by playing a variety of sports. She believes that if you can take control of your body, then you can be in control of other events in your life. However, she concludes, "The main way I take care of myself is though my faith."

Diane believes that soul represents the spiritual essence of a person. "It may be my Catholic belief system," she says, "but I believe we are born with a soul. We both enhance and build it up through our life experiences or we can damage and even destroy it by what we fail to do. A nurse connected to soul will speak about the emotional needs of patients as well as their clinical situation and may use holistic activities such as healing touch, prayer, and other therapies. I believe soul becomes enhanced when we embrace empathy and ask the question, 'What would I want if I were in that bed?'"

Diane is often assigned the more difficult patients. She explained, "For example, I had a woman who had a heart condition and who was also eight months pregnant. She had been in the hospital for four months because they didn't think she would be able to carry the pregnancy through birth. She was a very angry woman. It was difficult at first to get past her verbal attacks, but the more I got to work with her, the more her underlying fear began to come to the surface. Finally, she let me enter her emotional space and connect. That is what I mean by connecting with soul, getting underneath the surface."

Diane believes that maintaining belief represents one of the fundamental processes of caring. Accordingly, she identified *conviction* as one of her most valued skill clusters. One of her main goals as a nurse is to promote this form of caring. There is always hope, even when there doesn't appear to be any hope. It stems from a belief in a Higher Being or Power. Diane states, "I try to share this with my patients. I don't use the word *God* or specify the nature of this Higher Power unless it is appropriate. However, it is important to attempt to transmit that there is reason to hope. Of course, this doesn't usually happen in one interaction, and certainly I don't want to give any false hope. Basically, I want people to know that I am here for them."

At one point in her career, Diane experienced considerable burnout. Working in a cardiac care unit was both fatiguing and frustrating when she was not able to care for the patients with the kind of depth and focus she desired. "I eventually left to become a utilization review nurse, believing that I might be able to help patients to get extended care and better treatment by working with the insurance companies and the like. But what eventually brought me back to direct clinical care were the people and the realization that I could make a difference in their lives. Recently, I had the opportunity to work with a man who was very depressed and beyond hope in terms of living. I was privileged to listen to what he had to say. As I left his room, I thought to myself, this is why I am a nurse. I made a difference in this person's life this evening."

Continuing, she affirms, "Even with all the turmoil and chaos during these difficult times, I remain in health care because I know that I am making a difference, not only with my patients and their families, but within the system and with the other employees. Another reason I returned to the floor involved the wonderful nurses with whom I work. There is a deep sense of camaraderie and purpose working together as a team because we make a conscious effort to understand and to help one another."

Diane finds that often the grieving process is a communal affair and it often deepens staff relationships. As such, the staff utilizes rituals to ease the tension. She affirms, "It goes back to the fact that we work together and know each other so well. This is especially true during a code. We know whose job it is to do whatever is required. At the end of a code, we support each other and provide positive feedback. I don't know if there is any one specific ritual, but there are probably many of them involved in the routines of the day. And, if the person has passed away, we take the time to talk and cry together. Also, we have a hands-on supervisor, a person who participates to the 'doing' as well as the leading."

Diane's "You can do it!" passion underscores her desire to be a patient's cheer-leader, an attitude we view as being vitally important to the *enabling* aspect of the caring process. Diane states, "I always like to leave my patients with the idea that, regardless of the situation, they can do some things for themselves. Sometimes people, and especially those with a debilitating illness, become depressed and give up too much of their power and that tends to create codependency. So, I attempt to help patients identify and to engage in activities over which they do have control."

Diane tells the story about one of her patients, a 24-year-old diabetic man who loved to run. "Diabetics can be slow to heal, and this man was bitten on the toe by a spider," she relates. "They tried to save his toe, but could not do it and had to amputate his foot. When I walked into his room, one of the first things he said to me was, 'I've lost my foot, but I still have my leg.'"

She concludes, "Such experiences feed my soul and bring joy to my life and work." As we have seen, for Diane, joy also involves bringing a heart-filled presence to nursing, embracing challenge, and seeking the good and the beautiful in every experience.

# COMPASSIONATE CATALYST

## Susan Huntley, RN
### *Clinical nurse: Enabling energy to flow*

Colville is nestled in northeastern Washington amid some of the state's most scenic countryside. It is where we find the Healing Arts Center and Sue Huntley, RN.

Lon Hatfield, MD, opened the Healing Arts Center in 1998. With a twinkle in his eye, Lon confesses that he is a "recovering physician." Explaining, he states, "For me, a lot of allopathic medicine just doesn't work, and letting go of that some years ago to start a new program was a huge undertaking." Sue works as Lon's office nurse three days a week. The Center offers a holistic approach to health care, purporting that anyone who has an illness can effectively draw upon his or her physical, mental, social, emotional, and spiritual strengths to help regain his or her health.

Sue was born and raised in Metaline Falls, about 50 miles northeast of Colville and about 10 miles from the Canadian border. Upon graduating from nursing school, she joined the staff of the small Metaline Falls hospital where her mother, also a nurse, was the administrator. When the hospital found it could not afford to continue upgrading its medical equipment as mandated by new government regulations and closed, Sue tried school nursing. She later joined Lon's staff and embraced his approach to health care.

She states, "During the last 20 years, the word *holistic* has grown in use relative to health care. The allopathic medical community does a really good job of treating the body for acute situations. It is effective and it deserves its current recognition and support. However, we humans have physical, emotional, psychological, and spiritual dimensions. If one of these dimensions is neglected, the rest of them will be negatively impacted. Therefore, to be effective caregivers, holistically, we need to address every aspect of personhood."

Continuing, she reflects, "The more I speak with people, the more I see symptoms resulting from some underlying process. This is affirmed by Carolyn Myss, who asserts that biography often becomes biology. Biographical events leave biological imprints. We are one and the same with our life and our history. Events that have not yet been reconciled, forgiven, or released are carried as debt in cell tissue. For example, suppose some young punk comes up behind you and slaps you painfully on the back of the head while you are walking down the street eating an apple. The memory of that traumatic event and its negative emotions become attached to the act of eating an apple and may reoccur when again eating an apple. We may not even be consciously aware of it, because at least 75% of all communication occurs non-verbally." She further explains that some people may have a genetic predisposition to being allergic to apples, though the allergy may not be manifested physically until triggered by negative emotions.

This is one reason why Sue trained to become certified in a treatment process called Nambudripad's Allergy Elimination Technique (NAET). You can read about it at www.NAET.com. It is a safe, effective, natural approach to detecting and eliminating all types of allergies. NAET combines techniques from kinesiology (muscle strength testing), chiropractic, and Oriental medicine to clear allergic reactions through a "reprogramming" of the brain.

Sue explains, "Chinese medicine describes 12 major meridians; they are channels running deep in the tissues of the body and through them flows an invisible energy that the Chinese call 'life force.' It is the energy residing in and between our cells as described by quantum physics. Think of each meridian as being a river. Each one of these rivers may contain a dam, representing an allergy. For example, the dam may be an allergy to eggs. NAET rebalances the flow of energy through a chiropractic technique of applying light acupressure along both sides of the spinal column. If you could see this energy flowing into your body, it would enter through the top of your head and down through your spine to nerve roots. The task involves keeping the channel open from obstructions so the energy may flow. Illness occurs when there is a blockage of this energy anywhere along the pathways."

As an NAET practitioner, Sue works to rebalance the river of energy by removing the dam (the allergen). If you have a dam in the river, water backs up, or in our case, energy backs up, creating symptoms of illness. At the same time, downstream from the dam, not enough energy gets into the systems. That also creates symptoms. The dam is removed through the rebalancing process, which involves massaging along the back of the body. A new message is sent to the brain and to every cell in the body, because every cell acts like a computer chip storing memory. It informs the cells that the negative reaction is no longer necessary.

"Because of my faith system as a Roman Catholic, I tend to be skeptical of 'weird' practices and philosophies," she recounts. "On the other hand, I embrace a universe that is ultimately mysterious. So, I had to not dismiss NAET at first, but work through my thoughts about it. In addition, I pray every time I begin an NAET process. I know that whatever happens through this treatment is coming from God through my physical, mental, spiritual, and emotional presence. This is how I am able to integrate this methodology with my faith.

"I really came to integrate this belief into my work when my mother developed colon cancer. Being nurses, both she and I had administered various chemotherapy drugs to patients. When it was time for her to take these medications, her brain had a memory of them. The issue became whether she was sensitive to them. We used NAET to test her and to treat her for allergic reactions before she began taking the drugs.

"A few of the drugs were new to both of us. They were described on paper. My mother put her hand on the paper, and her senses were able to pick up the energy from the words. What this taught me, among other things, is that if there is that much energy in the environment, it is no wonder that so many people, kids in particular, have such difficulties. Apart from being surrounded by harmful chemicals, kids are exposed to all kinds of abuse, negativity, violence, and the like."

Because we also perceive soul as an underlying, mysterious web of energy, we asked Sue to describe her understanding of soul. She reports, "If you had asked me that 20 years ago, I would have answered differently. To me, soul was what we humans had. Other creatures and things did not have a soul. However, today my understanding is that everything has a soul. I identify life energy with soul. What differentiates human beings from other forms of life is that we have the spirit of God in our soul. It is the Imago Dei, the image of God. Trees that have life have soul, but do not have spirit. Soul leaves when a person or thing dies, but in a human, the spirit lives on throughout eternity."

| Skill Clusters | Transferable Skills |
|---|---|
| Compassion | Understanding/Tact |
| Conviction | Using Experience |
| Self-directing | Persuading |
| Communication | Advising |
| Flexibility | Emotional Control |
| Analytical | |
| Learning | |

It is no surprise that one of Sue's key skill clusters is *conviction*. She comments, "Working in a hospital for 18 years, I saw a lot of people dying. During this period, Elizabeth Kubler-Ross wrote about pioneering research relative to the grief process. It was very helpful, because coming from the Christian tradition, I always believed there was something out there called Eternity. Helping people make this transition so they weren't afraid represents a skill that comes with time and experience. For example, I am currently in a situation where I am caring for a baby who will not live to be more then two years old because she has a genetic disorder. Part of what I am doing with the family involves helping the 20-year-old mother learn about the grieving process and come to a point of acceptance. The baby is going to die; how do you want this to take place? Do you want this to occur at home, or do you want to prolong life as long as possible at a hospital in Spokane? I am helping this mother make some painful decisions. At the same time, it is important for me to be an advocate for the baby, who can't speak for herself because she is only 13 months old. From a nursing viewpoint, I know what the options are, but as an advocate for the child, I ask, what is best for her? I believe that it is important to love and care for the child, have a supportive environment, and keep her as pain free as possible."

Sue further explains, "We went through this with my mother. She was at home dying with cancer and, along with my sister [also a nurse] and my other siblings, we took turns caring for her. Actually, it was a beautiful experience lasting for about three weeks. We wondered at the time why we were being so blessed. She had her feet in both worlds for a period. She would talk to God, Jesus, and the Blessed Mother and then inform us what was happening. Some skeptics would say it was all her imagination, but we could feel a mysterious presence. The last few hours were difficult, but we were available to do what needed to be done."

It is quite possible that without being conscious of it, in her own way with her own agenda, Sue's mother was utilizing some of her finest, most cherished nursing skills during the last few weeks of her life. Nursing professor Patricia Donahue reminds us, "Nursing is not merely a technique but a process that incorporates the elements of soul, mind, and imagination."

Imagination is a technique that has been available since the dawn of history. When the Swiss psychologist Carl Jung began practicing it, he called it "active imagination." Although it requires discipline and hard work, stated simply, it involves visualization and placing oneself imaginatively into a particular scene or event. For example, when talking to Jesus, Sue's mother may have been visualizing herself present with Jesus and the disciples on the Sea of Galilee or at the Last Supper.

Another one of Sue's skill clusters relates to *compassion,* and from listening to her, it became apparent that it weaves its way throughout the tapestry of her work. It especially involves understanding and empathizing, or walking in another person's shoes. As such, we wondered how she avoids burnout. She comments, "It is a process that I have had to learn over the years. For the first 25 years, it seemed as though energy was going out from me but not much was coming back. I eventually faced burnout; this is why I will not work in a hospital again. It's too high-tech and too stressful. I engage in nursing on a more low-key, home health, and clinic basis. As I remain connected with people, I find it very rewarding."

Considering her life retrospectively, Sue hopes others will say at its end "that I loved people and made an effort to see the good in everyone." As such, a motto for her life and work might be "Compassionate catalyst for positive and holistic change." She reminds us, "Of course, because I am human, I do dislike certain attitudes and actions. I especially dislike behaviors associated with being a martyr. However, I find myself believing that God puts such people in my path for a purpose, and I work to find the good in them. I really enjoy looking for this goodness. I'm not naive enough to believe that anyone is perfect, but I believe there is the spirit of God within all people."

# FELLOW SOJOURNER

### Joan E. Purdon, MSN, CS, RN
*Parish nurse: Nursing spirituality*

Joan Purdon finds health ministry to be some of the most rewarding work she has done. It allows her to take the knowledge and skills gained from a 30-year nursing career and integrate them with her faith-based Christian beliefs assisting people to move from one level of health to another. "On an everyday basis, I am able to synthesize nursing and spirituality," she says warmly.

Joan wanted to be a nurse from the time she was very young. An aunt was in the Army Nurse Corps and rose through the ranks to become a lieutenant colonel. "As a rare independent career woman in the 1950s and 1960s, she was a role model. She encouraged and inspired me. When I entered high school, I became a candy striper," she recalls. "My dad was a Lutheran minister, and I often went with him on Sunday afternoons to the hospital while he visited the sick. I remember enjoying just sitting in the lobby and soaking up the hospital atmosphere while he made his rounds," she laughs.

Early on, Joan was especially drawn to nursing education. In the beginning, she worked as a pediatric staff nurse for about 15 years as she raised her family. However, she always knew that she would eventually return to school to become a nurse educator. In 1983, she entered graduate school and later worked for 15 years at the University of Cincinnati Raymond Walters College, Associate Degree Program in Nursing. Moving to Atlanta, she taught part-time at Kennesaw State University School of Nursing.

"I had known about parish nursing for a period of time and began to read some books on the subject," she remembers. "I was drawn to this ministry and wanted to explore it in more depth. So, I entered a parish nursing preparation course. As part of my community service and call to parish nursing, I instituted, and for four years actively participated in, a volunteer parish nursing program at my home church."

When her husband's work and the desire to be closer to family precipitated a move to Atlanta, her previous parish nursing volunteer experience served as preparation for her current work. Shortly after the move, Joan says gratefully, "I received a wonderful gift! There was an opening to be a parish nurse in a large congregation.

Here I am able to draw on everything from the time I received my nurse's license in 1970, including my general life experiences," she affirms enthusiastically. Today, she serves as the Director of Health Ministries, St. Luke's Episcopal Church, Atlanta, and Saint Joseph's Hospital Mercy Care Services.

Joan's faith is the basis of her understanding of the meaning of soul and spirituality. "There is spirit in each one of us, linking us to all of humanity and to our Creator," she believes. "It becomes a part of our inner being, yet transcends our bodies. Spirituality is a mysterious concept being expressed in many different ways—through your relationships, through nature, music, art, and work. There exists a spirituality that is not necessarily religious. Our home backs up to a lake, so nature surrounds us. For the first time, I can walk to it anytime I wish; it revives my soul. One of my spiritual practices is to connect each day to nature in some way. Practices like these keep me grounded and strong, so when I meet people in need, I can be present and caring, helping them on their journeys."

Two books have been important influences on her work: *The Healing Presence*[3] (1992) by Thomas Droege, a series of scriptural-based meditations, and *Spirituality in Nursing: Standing on Holy Ground*[4] (2003) by Mary Elizabeth O'Brien. The latter book manages to touch all of the important bases, she believes, beginning with a spiritual history of nursing and quickly moving on to a nursing assessment of spiritual needs relative to various life stages. Joan particularly relates to the idea of walking on holy ground when in the presence of a patient.

The use of prayer is a significant part of health ministry, according to Joan. "Let me explain with an example," she continues, "I currently work with an individual who is in the latter stages of cancer. Therapy is not helping, and the tumor continues to grow. I was present when this individual received the bad news and had to consider possible alternatives. We met again a few days later after this individual decided to terminate therapy. All of these interactions include a prayer component, asking for strength. They are part of the process of helping someone accept where they are in their journey."

She confesses, "Interestingly, at the beginning of my work as a parish nurse, I was less comfortable with praying with a person, just letting the words come forth. I could not have done this when I was in my twenties or thirties."

In yet another story demonstrating healing, she tells the story of a woman without health insurance who came to her after having a mastectomy and losing her job. She needed help to find a support group and money to live on while searching for new employment. Joan reports, "I was able to refer her to an appropriate support group, obtain food from a local organization, and solicit a no-interest loan from the pastor's discretionary fund. Since then, this woman found a job, has become active in the parish, and recently completed a small group facilitator-training program. So, she has come full circle from being a person in great need to serving others."

Promoting preventative health care is yet another component of Joan's work. She coordinates a Day Timer's Health Promotion program. Designed to reach senior citizens, this group meets monthly to learn about such subjects as preventing falls, osteoporosis, disaster preparedness, nutrition, and heart health.

While the context of the word *caring* is difficult to describe briefly, we asked Joan to explore its meaning with us. For her, it means to meet people where they are at any particular moment, to listen, and to place one's personal agenda aside. Often there is no way to fix the problem, she notes, so in these situations a caring moment is simply being mindfully present. She places particular attention upon the *being with* process of caring. To be fully present in the moment involves processing the dynamics of the relationship without focusing on what to say next, honoring the other person's expressions, not making assumptions, and recognizing the value of the person's context and culture.

At the same time, we know that a patient's perception of a caring moment may differ from that of the caregiver. For many patients, caring means accessibility, close monitoring of their situation, following through on promises, and recognizing individual needs. But again, for both nurse and patient, caring involves being present in the moment and listening.

| Skill Clusters | Transferable Skills |
|---|---|
| Maximizing | Training |
| Learning | Advising |
| Analytical | Potential Problem-solving |
| Compassion | Drive/Tenacity |
| Leadership | Serving |
| Managerial Competence | |
| Service/Dedication | |

Joan utilizes her skill cluster of *maximizing* by giving people considerable encouragement, which especially involves "going the distance with people." She often uses similar phrases such as "I'm going to journey along with you." "It means that I will not leave or abandon you in this process," she says firmly. "This is especially true with people facing a terminal illness or other grief issues. I express confidence that they can find a way to work through the situation and do not have to go it alone. I serve as their advocate particularly in terms of uncovering appropriate resources."

Her *learning* and *analytical* skill clusters especially relate to the *knowing* aspect of providing care. As an intuitive, "big picture" person, she wants to know how an individual fits into a family system, the parish, and to other life connections. "It involves capturing one's story, from whence you come," she says warmly. "I always like to say, 'Tell me more about that.' Once I know a person's story, it becomes easier to help him or her; it's the compassion piece of the puzzle. It allows us to move to the next step of *doing for*, and nurses are especially good doers and fixers," she smiles.

"However, in health ministry, often we can't fix things, but we can help people to obtain the resources. That is where *compassion* enters the picture, the ability to accept what someone says even though it may be ugly and painful. I am currently assisting a man who over the past few years spoke often about his smoking. He takes blood pressure medication. After taking his blood pressure as requested, I told him that he knew what to do to help the situation. He said, 'Yes, quit smoking!' So, the door opened to journey with him in the process of change. I didn't approach him a few years earlier with 'shoulds and oughts,' but waited for a compassionate opportunity to arise. Much of my work today entails building a relationship of trust. This is very different from many other nursing situations, where you see patients for a limited period of time, especially in acute care or outpatient settings. I see people many, many times."

Joan's *leadership* and *managerial competence* especially came to play when for eight years she was chair of the Nursing Department at the University of Cincinnati, Raymond Walters College. Her basic job was creating a vision and, again, using her intuition to see the big picture, trusting that her colleagues had the competency to perform the work.

We especially wanted to ask about her skill of *drive/tenacity*. "First, I must say that I have learned to take care of myself," she exclaims. "In high school, I was a straight 'A' student, a leader in many organizations and very active in church groups. I also loved working in the library because I enjoy a scholarly orientation. It became easy to overextend myself! Because of that, my mother taught me a very early lesson to set priorities. My sense of drive also comes forth in terms of giving my best to any involvement."

Today, Joan takes care of herself by limiting her parish work to 20 hours per week and by teaching on a part-time basis. She exercises and walks each day, maintaining the connection with nature, the love of which came from her father. "Care for yourself first," she admonishes. "So often, nurses don't do a very good job of that, although we are probably getting better at it. You have to know yourself well enough, your abilities and limitations, to be able to care for others."

# I Can Do That!

## Dee Lowe Horn, RN
### *Home care nurse: Enterprising up-front organizer*

I f Dee Lowe Horn were given a tee shirt with a slogan that sums up her philosophy of life, it might read, "I Can Do That!" With her vast array of interests and talents, ranging from an extensive and varied nursing career to belly dancing, playing the flute, photography, and winning blue ribbons for her canning and bread making to her newest endeavor, designing jewelry, she embodies someone unafraid of trying new opportunities. Perhaps because she is sensitive to life's fleeting moments, she embraces whatever interests her at the moment.

Her career in nursing began as a candy striper in a geriatric hospital. She remembers fondly, "They gave me a gold charm that was a nurse's cap and said that I needed to enter nursing because it appeared to be my calling." She did not respond to that calling until later, however. "After finishing school, I found a secretarial job in a hospital. I could not help but become involved with some of the patients, so I began taking nursing classes and graduated in 1982 from Southwestern College in San Diego."

Her nursing career spans a dozen years in critical care as an emergency, flight, and ambulance nurse, to becoming a nursing supervisor in a home care agency in Salt Lake City. Not happy with the lack of direct patient contact, she subsequently returned to more hands-on patient care.

Dee believes that home care is the heart and soul of nursing. She finds it to be a good arena for her organizational and nursing skills, viewing it as the best opportunity to use a wide array of nursing skills, especially the human relations aspect. She avows, "It's the opportunity to be in a person's home for five minutes or five hours, depending upon their needs and my schedule. In a hospital, you simply do not have the time and flexibility. I enjoy following up on a treatment plan and seeing people progress. I like looking at people's homes, their art and pictures; it helps me connect with them. I rely on my nursing intuition in looking at people and being able to assess them without their saying a word. Plus," she says, "in home care, I am not in charge. The patient is in charge. In the home, the nurse is asking permission to enter the patient's life, asking to perform a procedure, not telling her or him what to do." Dee likes empowering people to make decisions. Even when scheduling an appointment, she asks if it is convenient. "In the hospital," she explains, "patients tend to be very compliant and dependent upon someone else's schedule and whim and feel that that they are not in control. Of course," she underscores, "patients really are in control in the hospital, but they don't feel that way because the environment is so overwhelming."

| Skill Clusters | Transferable Skills |
| --- | --- |
| Creativity | Training |
| Accountability | Using Experience |
| Service/Dedication | Innovating |
| Technical Competence | Drive/Tenacity |
| Entrepreneurship | Dependability |
| Compassion | |
| Visionary | |

One of Dee's specific, satisfying skills involves *training* and includes the ability to translate a technical issue or procedure into patient-friendly language. Some patients might say, "There is no way I can learn this," like self-administering an antibiotic. However, Dee excels in helping others overcome their initial resistance through her ability to teach, passing on her own "I can do that" philosophy. In fact, she views teaching as a major focus of home care, empowering people to become more independent, thus enabling them to become more self-reliant and less dependent upon hospitals and healthcare professionals.

Dee's delight in training and teaching was apparent as an Emergency Department nurse. "We get a lot of children coming into the ED and that can be a frightening experience for a child, not knowing what to expect." So, as part of a patient advocacy program, she made a video taken from a child's eye level with the camera becoming the child. The scenario followed a child who enters the ED with a cut that requires stitches. Dee later took the video into local elementary schools, speaking to kindergarten through 4th grade classes, teaching children to be less fearful of a potential ED visit. She showed them all of the objects associated with treatment—gowns, oxygen masks, needles, and the like—that they might see. After viewing the video, they had an opportunity to ask questions. The project is just one of many examples of Dee's creativity.

Dee's priority skill cluster is *creativity*. She reports, "I am always looking for some way to make it easier for people to be able to meet their needs and improve procedures. For example, I developed an IV supply reference guide for my pharmacy department and IV patients. The guide allows patients to call a product by its name, understand how it is used, and easily order a refill over the telephone. It's hard to communicate clearly by someone asking for more of that 'little pink thing or that round thing,'" she laughs. "In nursing, I am always attempting to find a way to make life easier or more pleasant."

Dee tells the story of a tourist from Central America who was visiting relatives in Salt Lake City. "She was riding in a car when an accident occurred. Her uncle and cousin were killed and the woman became a quadriplegic. She didn't speak any English yet she had to be quickly integrated into a system that could not help her because she had no insurance or money. The United Way supports our agency," Dee explains, "so I went in to the home to teach the mother how to care for her. They had no idea how they were going to get the necessary supplies. I happened to know of an agency that disperses money from an anonymous donor. I contacted them and then convinced local vendors to donate items or contribute additional supplies at a lower cost. What I did involved resourcing, knowing whom to contact, and convincing them to help. If you tell a story of legitimate need, people want to help because we work in a very caring, empathetic, and loving profession," she says firmly.

It's no surprise that another of Dee's key skills entails *drive/tenacity*. She never gives up and has never done so throughout her life. She remains persistent in uncovering resources and enlisting people to help. She declares, "I've always been a person who goes for the gold. I do it even beyond nursing." Sharing her latest venture, she admits that without previous experience, she started a new business making jewelry. "I had to locate all the vendors and get everything organized. Now I have a bookkeeper, a buyer, and an assistant. All of this occurs because I talk to people, getting to know them and not being afraid to put myself on the line. I believe that when one door closes, another door opens."

Today, Dee maintains a caseload of over 100 patients, with about 50% of her time spent in direct patient care, which requires prioritizing and being organized. Her ability to store and recall a great quantity of information is critical. She also knows how to persuade people, getting people to do things for her, making them feel good about it. Again, it's her philosophy of "I can do that!"

Dee describes soul as the essence of nursing. "It's *why* we care, not in a technical sense, but holding a hand, crying with a patient, letting him or her know that I understand his or her pain." She remains committed to nursing because of an ability to make people feel good and to help them cope with their problems. She especially enjoys teaching people how to manage their situation and how to participate in getting well again.

She informs us, "For example, with pain problems, I teach people how to not allow the pain to get control of them. I especially believe in positive thinking. I have had thousands of patients, but I remember one gentleman back in 1982 when I was an orthopedic nurse. Doctors just started using medication for herniated discs. They were injecting papaya into the disc to eat away at it. Back then, you might stay in the hospital for weeks on end. I was preparing this man for surgery and he said, 'You know, I'm going home within a day after surgery.' I told him that never happens. He replied that it can make an enormous difference if you have positive thoughts. I laughed, but when I returned to work the second day after surgery, he had been released from the hospital."

Dee believes that by working on the positive side of energy flow, people will heal more quickly. "Humor also helps," Dee says. "I believe that is why my patients like me, because I am a funny person. I go to their homes and laugh with them. I tie this back to holistic nursing. Whatever the therapies, such as the use of herbs or healing touch, it is a matter of embracing anything that makes someone feel better."

We view Dee as someone who has many gifts to give her patients—from teaching and offering encouragement to positive thinking. We asked her to share what she sees as her a primary gift. "I think it's compassion," she responds quickly. "It's my putting myself in their situation. How would I want to be treated if I were lying in that bed and could not get out of it? I teach home health aides that, before leaving a place, put yourself mentally in that bed and look around. Do you have water, access to a phone, and entertainment so that you are not staring at the walls? Are you warm enough and positioned correctly?"

She views herself as a high-energy person who, in addition to nursing and other activities, still finds time to volunteer. Her lifetime of volunteering generally involves fun, such as pouring beer at a local arts festival. Asked how she takes care of herself, she quickly responds, "By doing all of my fun things; I try not to take work home with me. I may think about what I need to do for someone, but I don't let it drag me down emotionally. If I am compromised, I can't help another person."

Dee confesses that she wears her heart on her sleeve. She reports that people who know her say that she "tells it like it is." This trait, together with her ability to clinically and passionately care for her patients, plus her considerable resourcing talents and motivational skills, undoubtedly led to her inclusion since 1993 in *Who's Who in American Nursing*.

# Connecting Through Competence and Compassion

### Carolyn Spence Cagle, PhD, RNC
*Nursing professor: Change agent*

With two aunts who were nurses as role models, it is no surprise that Carolyn Cagle, professor of nursing at Texas Christian University's College of Health and Human Sciences, became a nurse. She attributes her close relationship with them as a driving factor in her career choice. "They were both nurses, so I grew up with a positive image of the profession. For me, providing care to people bestows a kind of internal energy propelling you through life," she states. "One of my aunts was a psychiatric nurse; the other worked in critical care."

Neither of her aunts' chosen specialties particularly interested Carolyn, however, and eventually she became attracted to pediatrics. She finds working with new families who are excited about their babies rewarding, and she thoroughly enjoys helping people become quality parents. Maternity has long been a real love for Carolyn, although her teaching and research have broadened beyond maternity topics. Helping young families become healthier represents a big part of her orientation. Both professionally and personally, she understands that giving birth to a child is much more than a physical phenomenon; it involves one's emotional and spiritual self as well. At the time of this interview, she herself was in the middle stages of child rearing.

According to Carolyn, an internal core or energy drives her passion for nursing. She is especially drawn toward parenting her children and volunteering with health-care-related organizations such as the American Heart Association. On and off the job, she enjoys creating teams of people who work together. "I enjoy getting faculty connected to administration so a common vision can emerge."

When the university recently decided to revise the core curriculum, Carolyn became involved as chair of the Faculty Senate, leading that group in the process and serving as a liaison with university officials involved in core discussions. "It was quite a challenge, but I think it was quite a good process for everyone. In fact, we are still continuing that work. It was exciting for me to be outside of nursing per se and to serve as a faculty advocate. The process taught me a lot about how I respond to difficulties and challenges," she explains.

She admits that achieving a common vision is not an easy task, "However, this is who I am and what I do well, what feeds my soul. In the frenzy of life, the connections between people through committed listening and other effective communication skills often simply don't happen."

| Skill Clusters | Transferable Skills |
|---|---|
| Conviction | Enlisting |
| Leadership | Questioning |
| Achievement-oriented | Conveying Emotions |
| Service/Dedication | Negotiating |
| Relating | Drive/Tenacity |
| Acceptance | |
| Connectivity | |

Reviewing Carolyn's skills and listening to her speak about her passion leads us to suggest that she might thrive as an organizational development (OD) professional, a person who helps create organizational vision and systematically assists in shaping an environment to achieve desired results. She enjoys challenging the status quo, using her skills of *drive/tenacity* and *questioning*. Her skill cluster of *conviction*, steadily maintaining a core set of beliefs and values, blends well with the university's stated mission of ethical leadership and global citizenship.

Carolyn especially likes conducting qualitative research, looking at the context of a situation. "For example," she reports, "I submitted a grant to study how the work environment supports or detracts from the health care of women. It includes researching what it is like to go to work every day, having very limited control." She speculates, "What is it like to have very limited or no healthcare coverage, but needing to work in order to survive? Then when you add a chronic illness to the situation, how do people in general, and women in particular, cope from day to day? They just do it, but end up dying at age 55. Our healthcare system simply does not ethically address people who face such issues. Most of the leaders of our healthcare system in this country prefer to relate to people who share similar values, especially in terms of the bottom-line and money."

Moving from clinical hospital nursing to a career in academia grew out of her desire to improve the quality of nursing. She explains, "I became committed to helping people become better nurses. I want my students to understand the value of having a caring attitude along with a competent knowledge base, bringing such elements to improve a workforce. Here at the college, the feedback we receive suggests that we do this quite well." However, with concern she states, "It is becoming increasingly difficult to maintain these values because of the shortage of qualified nursing professors and an unclear idea of how to focus on priorities. So often, we must rely upon adjunct faculty who work part time and who have limited ability to access and contribute to the college's overall mission. This dilutes our services."

Carolyn maintains that many nursing educators get their satisfaction from the "high-tech" side of the equation. While balancing the two, it is not surprising that she commits more energy to "high touch." "I think you have to balance the two," she states. She cares for her students by using her skill clusters such as *acceptance* and *relating*, which are linked to the caring processes of *knowing* and *being with*. "I don't take on the burdens of the students I advise, but I am with them in their learning. As the old adage suggests, 'Inch by inch is a cinch—yard by yard is hard.' I want them to frame things in the context of something that is easy to do, with a focus on the content of the day. All of this content adds up by week's end to a great deal of learning." Through her *service* and *dedication,* she enables students to excel in their education.

On a more personal level, Carolyn's *teaching* and *negotiating* skills coupled with her enabling style were instrumental in helping her mother cope with her father's home recuperation following a heart attack. "My father, who had always been healthy," she explains, "had a heart attack three years ago, which destroyed a third of his heart muscle. My mother didn't want to hear the term congestive heart failure. When I went to visit, I helped her to develop a list of things to watch for. The charting activity helped my mother become more independent and also generated positive feedback from his physician."

Competence and collaboration stand among Carolyn's core values. Collaboration involves an understanding that each party involved in a procedure or project is very important to the outcome. "It all balances out," she affirms. "It becomes a win-win situation, making the outcome and the organization so much stronger. Unfortunately, often I find myself being a kind of maverick and being in the minority in this respect. My strongly held values have made my jobs in several workplaces challenging at times, but ultimately I believe my actions will make a difference in improving those work settings."

Thinking out of the box is one of Carolyn's key skills, closely related to her maverick attitude. She is able to question assumptions and perceptions. Some inventions and adaptations are functional and serve us well, but obviously in today's chaotic healthcare environment, reformation has become essential.

Collaboration and her skill cluster of *connectivity* stand side by side. She believes that everything is connected and has purpose. She affirms, "We may not know the significance of an event when it happens, but over time, understanding begins to surface."

Carolyn views Parker Palmer as one of her heroes. His book *The Courage to Teach*[5] (1999) is based on the premise that "good teaching cannot be reduced to technique; good teaching comes from the identity and integrity of the teachers." Palmer examines some of the reasons for teacher isolation and fragmented systems, and he offers a guide to creating communities of learning and new feelings of wholeness. He suggests that only when we know ourselves can we help our students to develop into whole people who will become lifelong learners.

Palmer concludes, "when we are unfaithful to the inward teacher and to the community of truth, we do lamentable damage to ourselves, to our students, and to the great things of the world that our knowledge holds in trust . . . but if you are here faithfully with us, you are bringing abundant blessing. It is a blessing known to generations of students whose lives have been transformed by people who had the courage to teach."

Considering today's healthcare environment, Carolyn still recommends nursing to young people. "I would recommend nursing, if for no other reason than there are so many diverse opportunities," she says. "It is also a wonderful way to prepare for life in general. Nursing teaches you how to relate to other individuals, at least initially before becoming hard-core. There are also internal rewards of helping people to rediscover themselves and to grow. In addition, apart from the marriage relationship, nothing is more physically intimate than caring for someone who is ill or injured."

Continuing, she relates, "Increasingly, there is a lot more respect given to nurses compared with other professions. This provides one with an external reward as well. Nurses are becoming more and more empowered, often being health care's gatekeepers. As nurses become more comfortable in providing education, going beyond technology, respect for the profession will continue to escalate. For this reason, we teach our students to go beyond the obvious, not just taking blood pressures but also exploring other lifestyle choices. This is what makes for healthy individuals. So, the nurse is one person who can make all of the difference in terms of caring for people and helping them access the other pieces involved in health."

Carolyn is also optimistic about health care in general. "I'm optimistic," she states, "because I believe managed care will change considerably in the future. Consumers are infuriated about the services it provides. New paradigms will form. Also, the 40-plus million uninsured people in this country represent a powerful force for reform. It affects our productivity as a society, and if we don't take care of these people early on in life, then they become the liability of the future. So, there is food for optimism."

# ANYTHING'S POSSIBLE
## Sister Peggy Fannon, RSM, RN, CDE
### *Merciful patient educator*

The seeds for a life of caregiving were planted early, recalls Sister Peggy Fannon. "When I was four years old, I was hospitalized because of numerous ear infections. From that time on, all I ever talked about was being a nurse. As a young teen, I was inspired by the biographies of Florence Nightingale and Clara Barton. Then, there were the fictional adventures of Cherry Ames and Sue Barton," she said.

"As an older teenager," she continues, "I loved it when my mother shared stories about her parents. My maternal grandfather, who was a surgeon in the Spanish-American War, was William Howard Taft's personal physician when Taft was governor of the Philippines. He was later instrumental in starting the Catholic hospital in an Ohio town where he met my maternal grandmother, who was a nurse. Years later, I was born in the same hospital.

"My paternal grandmother was a tremendous influence in my life. My sister and I accompanied her on 'errands of mercy' as she visited sick friends, prepared and took food to their families, and even attended wake services of friends and loved ones. She would proudly tell her friends that I was going to be a nurse and a nun. I believe she planted and nurtured the seeds of my religious journey. Since several relatives were priests and nuns, sometimes I wonder if I inherited my vocation," she grins.

Sister Peggy's nursing career began before entering the Sisters of Mercy and spans 35 years in medical/surgical nursing, burn care, pediatrics, utilization review/discharge planning, and diabetes education. Her family moved to Atlanta when she was 11 years old. After high school graduation, she entered nursing school at the 346-bed St. Joseph's Hospital. The early years of nursing education and work were difficult ones that left painful and deep emotional memories. "My father died of a massive heart attack during my first year in training. Then, just before graduation, my mother was diagnosed with cancer and died two years later." Sister Peggy took over the role as head of household to raise her five younger brothers. "During this period, I was working as a staff nurse, as I took on both work and parenting responsibilities," she says. Gratefully, she gives testimony to the hospital's soulful and caring environment. This period in her life began her journey of living the "anything's possible" mantra.

As the children grew up and needed less supervision, Sister Peggy was increasingly drawn to church work, becoming involved in the Cursillo Movement,[6] a spiritual renewal movement sponsored by the Archdiocese of Atlanta. She explains, "I participated on the weekend teams by giving talks and performing other assigned duties that facilitated the weekend program. This ministry led to a deepened sense of my call from God. Following a year and a half of prayerful discernment and meetings with a spiritual director, I made the decision to go to Baltimore where I entered the Sisters of Mercy Community."

The Sisters of Mercy is an international religious community dedicated to serving God's people—especially those who are sick, poor, and uneducated. "The process of becoming a sister within this community takes about five to six years," she explains. Although a priest uncle advised Sister Peggy to explore other religious communities, "I knew this was the community for me," she states firmly. "I was taught by these Sisters in the grade and high schools I attended, as well as in the nursing school. Based upon my admiration for them and the ways they ministered to God's people, there was no question about my direction. After entering the community and taking final vows, I eventually returned to St. Joseph's Hospital in Atlanta."

Sister Peggy sees herself as serving in the arena of her passion and calling. As a Patient Education Specialist and Certified Diabetes Educator, she works mostly with inpatients suffering from diabetes. "Diabetes represents a growing health problem," she says warming to her subject. "There are roughly 17 million people walking around who don't even know they have a problem. Sometimes they enter the hospital with another problem before being diagnosed with diabetes." She works with patients who have had open heart surgery or a heart transplant and have diabetes as well. She also sees patients who have congestive heart failure or have experienced a heart attack and occasionally patients who have implantable devices, such as pacemakers or defibrillators.

"When I worked as a staff nurse and a manager, I personally never felt I had enough time to do all that was needed for my patients. So, after reporting off to the next shift, I usually stayed late addressing those needs. As a nurse educator, I have more flexibility with my time than I did in my earlier staffing assignments."

Sister Peggy views soul as the spiritual side or essence of a person and considers her work with patients as working with the "whole person." "For example," she explains, "when I worked on a nursing unit, some coworkers would point out that I always had the more difficult and needy patients. One such patient related that, while attending a private Catholic elementary school, he was accused unjustly of a wrongdoing by his teacher, a nun. The Sister reported this wrongdoing to his father, who severely punished the boy. Because of that experience, as an adult, he left the Church and gave up his faith. While under my care in the hospital, he confessed before he died that his whole perspective about Sisters had changed because of his encounter with me as his caregiver. To this day I am grateful to have provided him the opportunity to heal from an abusive religious and parental experience. His family was overjoyed at his peace."

St. Joseph's Hospital is different from secular hospitals because prayer is not foreign or discouraged, she notes. "When I worked on the oncology floor as a staff nurse and knew that someone needed more attention than I could give, I called for the Chaplain. However, I introduced myself to all my patients as 'Sister Peggy,' so they would know my background. Although I limited my role to nursing, at times I would pray with or discuss spiritual issues with my patients, if requested."

Continuing, she relates the following story. "Children develop trusting relationships more quickly than adults," she points out. "When I worked with children who had burn injuries, there was one little boy who found it quite difficult and painful to enter the whirlpool tub. Despite having been medicated prior to the treatment, the water would sting his open wounds for several seconds. To take his mind off of the sting as he was ready to enter the water, I would say, 'okay, let's say The Lord's Prayer together.' That helped him to focus on something other than his treatment."

| Skill Clusters | Transferable Skills |
| --- | --- |
| Service/Dedication | Enlisting |
| Compassion | Using Experience |
| Connectivity | Training |
| Flexibility | Serving |
| Maximizing | Synthesizing |
| Relating | |
| Technical Competence | |

*Maximizing* and *connectivity* serve as two of Sister Peggy's key skill clusters, especially as they apply to the caring process of *maintaining belief* in a healing outcome. "When I first approach people, I give them the benefit of the doubt," she states. "My basic orientation is nonjudgmental. I use my background and experience to explain the healing and recuperation processes and provide positive reinforcement of their progress made along the way. This underscores why *using experience* serves as one of my key transferable skills."

Reflecting, she informs us, "I find myself using a number of my key skills during a session with a patient. I certainly am *connecting* with people during a visit, using *compassion* while *enlisting* their cooperation and *training* them in the use of medications and procedures. I do all of this on a daily basis."

Her compassion in part springs from her personal journey. Over the years, she has shared her personal joys and sorrows with a number of patients and their families. "I believe it helps them to know something about my story," she affirms.

"I had a patient who was also a parishioner in our local church. After he left the hospital, there were times when I would visit him at home and provide essential care that was not being provided by the Home Health Agency. This also gave comforting support to his wife and family.

"When we had many children admitted for burn care at St. Joseph's Hospital, I often spent time with them after the dressing changes and wound care, reading stories and playing games to soften their perception of me as their nurse. Many hours were also spent with their parents for education and support.

"To this day," she relates, "I cannot leave a patient if I feel that something needs to be addressed beyond their physical needs. Recently, I had a patient who traveled to Atlanta because she had lost faith in the doctor who was treating her. When I walked into her room, she immediately began to cry. She had numerous issues that needed to be aired unrelated to her diabetes. I could not leave her when my duties were finished; its just part of who I am."

Going the extra mile for patients potentially could impact her own self-care, but Sister Peggy explains, "In recent years, I take a mini-vacation at least once each month. The Sisters of Mercy own a home in a beautiful setting used for retreat and relaxation purposes. I assist the Sister who maintains the property. I work 72 hours, so I have an extra day each pay period (twice a month)." In addition, I occasionally take short trips with my family. Also, each day I set aside time for prayer and meditation. I now live in an apartment by myself. I never lived alone before and I love it! It's nice sometimes to just 'be.' For me, self-care involves cultivating a relationship with my inner self, paying attention to the many clues that direct me purposefully and peacefully."

When asked what primary advice she would give to a new nurse just beginning her career, she said, "Begin with you. Self-care serves as a touchstone for the profession. Also," she emphasizes, "you need a sense of humor because so often we are dealing with life and death issues, especially in a hospital setting. Humor is part of working with people whom you enjoy."

Sister Peggy's long-time compassion and caring for her patients was honored by the hospital when she received the 2001 Ernest W. Franklin III Award for Nursing Excellence. Originally established in appreciation of the hospital's nursing staff, the award is given to individuals who represent the mission of the entire nursing staff and their dedication to excellence and compassion in the care of their patients. Reflecting on the award, she affirms, "My work has long been more of a ministry than a job to me. It is an honor for me to participate in the healing ministry of Jesus through my work here at St. Joseph's."

# ADVOCATE AT THE END OF LIFE
## Eve-lynn Civerolo, RN
### *Hospice nurse: Passion for helping others pass on*

Every journey is made easier if there is a guide who makes the trip alongside the traveler. As a hospice nurse, Eve-lynn Civerolo is that guide, helping her patients to die, hopefully to achieve peace, and sometimes to even experience joy in the process. Working steadfastly and quickly to develop a bond of trust, she often uses touch to help put people in a space where they know that she accepts whatever way they decide to venture down the pathway toward death.

"I view nursing as a calling," Eve-lynn affirms. "I can't imagine myself in any other profession. Nursing serves my heart and soul, especially working in hospice. Of course, over a 30-year career, I worked in several different specialty areas, with 13 of the past years being in hospice. Loving my work keeps me in the healthcare field. It is one of the major ways I have developed my spirituality, growth, and love for seeking out more knowledge of our transition after this phase of our existence," she states.

She recalls knowing from the age of six that she wanted to become a nurse. Born in Albuquerque, New Mexico, she eventually found her way to Maui, Hawaii. The climate fits her love of the outdoors, nature, and swimming. Agreeing that her name is unusual, she laughs and explains. "My mother was born in England where Evelyn is often used as a boy's name. She wanted to make it clear that it was a girl's name, so she inserted the hyphen and a second 'n.'"

Eve-lynn views soul as the essence of all of life. Although raised Roman Catholic, she finds even more meaning in Eastern spirituality and doesn't consider herself to be particularly religious. In her work as a nurse and in her own mental processes, East and West tend to be conjoined. "As a hospice nurse," she explains, "I tend to gravitate more toward Eastern traditions, because in the East, dying and death are likely to be integrated into people's lives, whereas in the West, we tend to push it away and deny it. Being so deeply connected with people in the dying process causes me to deepen my own spirituality in such orientations as Buddhism; today it serves more as the core of my being."

The concept of reincarnation was nowhere to be found in Roman Catholic theology when she was growing up, Eve-lynn reminds us. "But," she observes, "being at their bedside, I hear people telling about being visited by deceased family and friends. And, even in my own life, I experience feelings that I have been in a certain place before. I don't understand exactly how or in what manner, but I believe that life continues after death."

Eve-lynn's passion for her work shines through as she discusses her experiences with people who are nearing death, describing what it means, apart from the obvious need for pain management, to die in a peaceful manner. "During my many years working here at Hospice Maui," she says, "I have been fortunate because most of the people I have worked with have had beautiful deaths. By that, I mean there is a process somewhat similar to giving birth to a child. Like childbirth, people do go through a period of labor to get to a place where they seem to come to a kind of blissfulness. I have been at the bedside of many people who have been able to verbalize some kind of joy. With others, it's the look on their face that communicates harmony and ecstasy. There seems to be a sense of near total tranquility. I have seen this over and over again as I have been privileged to be with them at the time of their death, even with other family members surrounding them," she explains reminiscing.

Continuing softly, she recalls, "A very dear friend who was one of our hospice nurses allowed me to share her life during the time she was dying of cancer. Coming in and out of consciousness, she told of being in a space of incredible peace and beauty. You could see it in her face at certain times. At other times, her eyebrows would wrinkle as though she were working on some dark issue in her life. It is as though she were transitioning through the dark night of the soul, but when she came out of it she would often giggle, verbalizing that the trip was so beautiful that there were no words to describe its beauty and that she felt safe and loved.

"I also remember a young man who struggled, because when you are young, your body tends to remain strong. You may be ready to let go mentally and emotionally, but the body resists. His family remained with him and, at the end, was quite shaken by his moaning, which I believe was not a reaction to physical pain but possibly related to the process of letting go. The family wanted more morphine, but I asked him about it even though he was unconscious at the time. His eyes flew open and he said, 'I am *not* ready to let go.' He was in control, so we backed off and gave support to the family members. I believe he was working through some issue and didn't want the process to be terminated."

Eve-lynn calls this a process of reviewing one's life, of celebrating accomplishments, of grieving over mistakes and failures, of forgiving and of letting go. She tells us how amazing it can be. "You can enter the room one day to find that what was such a big issue previously is now done with and gone. And it happens on all levels—physical, emotional, spiritual."

For Eve-lynn, it becomes important to differentiate between physical, emotional, and spiritual suffering. To help people work through emotional and spiritual issues, the first objective is to eliminate physical pain; otherwise, no energy exists to deal with the other dimensions. She shares another story to illustrate. "I went to a patient's house one day in response to a frantic phone call from a man's family, stating that he was in terrible pain. Walking up the driveway from my car, I could hear him hollering. As I entered his room, I saw him lying on a hospital bed with his eyes closed, with no movement or restlessness, just a lot of yelling. He was all alone, as the family was all in another room where they could see him but were too distressed by his hollering to be by the bedside. I sat down beside him and said directly to him, 'Are you in physical pain?' He instantly stopped his hollering, opened his eyes, and said in a very loud voice, 'No!' Then he returned to his moaning. So, I went to his wife with whom he had been married for a long time and suggested that she not be afraid because he was not in physical pain. I suggested that she simply sit beside him for a while as a caring, loving presence. At which point he stopped his moaning and died that night.

"Here we may have had an example of someone working through a pain of the soul, but who was able to die peacefully in the presence of loved ones," she believes. "It's interesting because, at first, many people will tell you that they want to be left alone, but later they seem comforted by the presence of a caring person. It may be a relative, friend, or caregiver with whom they have established a close or intimate relationship. Or it could be just someone who can hold a safe space for allowing him or her to do his or her work undisturbed."

Eve-lynn believes that in order to assist people through the experience of their dying, it is helpful to have established a bond of trust with their caregivers. And, because most of the barriers and pretenses evaporate, that bond usually occurs quite rapidly. Also, people become very astute about whom they trust and confide in. "They can intuitively sense your state of mind and emotions when you come into their room. If you are fearful, they will know it. On the other hand, if you are open and willing to share their space, to listen and to be comfortable with their discomfort as well as your own, then they begin to bond. They will allow you to assist them, and by this, I simply mean holding a space for them in peace and love so they can work through their own grief. We do this by using a variety of techniques, everything from simply listening to therapeutic touch, reflexology, massage, and Reiki. I also incorporate material from the weeklong seminar I took on *Contemplative Care in Dying* with Dr. Joan Halifax, an anthropologist, author, and teacher at a Buddhist center in Santa Fe, New Mexico.

"Given the fact that you are totally present to the individual," Eve-lynn continues, "the sense of touch seems to be particularly welcome and effective with patients during certain phases in their dying. It connects your energy with the other person's energy field. I try to frame it in the context of that person's belief system. So, if an individual is a Christian, I speak or think in terms of the flow of energy from God. You could use Buddha, nature, prayer, or the universe in general as an image as you ask for this energy to flow through your hands during a touch or massage. For the people who are truly drawn to this touching therapy, it creates an aura of serenity."

Eve-lynn acknowledges that caring for herself in the midst of some deeply emotional experiences is critically important. "I have to work at it," she admits. "Sometimes I have a tendency not to be as compassionate with myself as with others," she sadly confesses. "I develop myself through my spiritual path, as well as through my love of being in nature and being near the water. In addition, meditation plays an important part of maintaining my well-being."

Eve-lynn's career path has not always been smooth. She experienced a significant setback a few years earlier when she served both as a hospice nursing supervisor and volunteer coordinator. She was asked to step down from her position because three of the eight nurses she supervised believed she was micromanaging them. "At first I was stunned," she admits," because no one told me there was a problem, so I was truly blind-sided. I kept working but also took time to assess my abilities and relationships. I thought about quitting hospice altogether," she states frankly, "but I quickly decided that this was only due to my own hurt ego—realizing I loved the work too much to leave it. I decided to keep the goals of hospice patient care in the forefront of my mind, leave supervision, and retain the volunteer coordinating work. It became the best decision I've ever made, and I never regretted it! I viewed this situation as a growth event, especially after working through the anger and resentment. I can now appreciate the diversity each coworker brings to this unique type of work. Almost every negative aspect of our lives can be turned into something positive," she says enthusiastically.

"This viewpoint was also influenced by the reality that my husband, Richard, had been diagnosed with lung cancer. My challenge, as well as growth in my work, has taken on a new dimension, what it is truly like to be on the other side of my work. Richard and I have firsthand experience in what it feels like to be the patient and family working through a loss. I cannot help but feel this personal hardship has only deepened my commitment to the work of our dying."

| Skill Clusters | Transferable Skills |
|---|---|
| Compassion | Conveying Emotions |
| Connectivity | Understanding/Tact |
| Service/Dedication | Flexibility |
| Self-directing | Drive/Tenacity |
| Accountability | Decision-making |
| Flexibility | |
| Historic | |

Our interview with Eve-lynn and the stories she shares reveal a very clear congruence with her skill clusters and transferable skills. We hear a woman who *connects* with her patients, exercising *compassion* and *understanding* without passing judgment. She allows and assists patients to make their transition as easy and meaningful as possible in their own way, while at the same time helping facilitate the grief and understanding of their loved ones. Her *flexibility* allows her to hold a space for her patients and their families, especially when it is uncomfortable, so a connection can be made at a higher level of truth. This is also what it means for her to be connected to soul and spirit.

Eve-lynn's skill of *drive/tenacity* serves to summarize her passionate calling to hospice. When people are dying, they are extremely vulnerable. They are going through the process of attempting to let go and to heal and do not have the energy to fight for what they really want. Some people know how they want to die and can even articulate it, but they look to the caregiver professional for validation and support. "For me, drive and tenacity have to do with patient advocacy," she states firmly. "I want desperately for individuals to have the death that they desire. Most people, including family, nurses, and doctors, have an agenda for a dying person about how they 'should' die. Whether acknowledged or not, death is such a big part of everyone's life that very strong agendas exist, even with people who deeply love the dying person. One of the most passionate things in my life involves helping people die the way they wish. I want to help everyone to learn what the patient wants at the end of life."

# LET'S GET BUSY!
## LOOKING FOR THE POSSIBLE

John Hanson, BS, RN

*Former Traveling Nurse: 23 countries, 32 states, 8 years*

Still in his thirties, John Hanson has traveled more and done more career-wise than many of us will do in a lifetime. While working at the King Faisal Specialty Hospital in Saudi Arabia, John and his wife, also a nurse, took many holidays traveling to other countries thanks to a generous time-off benefit given to foreigners to offset their cultural shock. In their three-and-a-half-year stay, they visited 23 different countries, fulfilling their primary goal of expanding their travel opportunities. Prior to their overseas work, both were traveling nurses in the United States and had visited 32 states. All of this took place in a period of only eight years. John affirms, "Many people don't recognize the opportunities available to nurses that exist in a variety of locations and nursing specialties."

Tongue in cheek, John inferred that he originally entered nursing because his wife was two years ahead of him in nursing school, and he thought he could copy her assignments, making it easier to get a degree. In reality, he admits, he has been associated with health care all of his life. "My mother was a certified nurse assistant, and if I was sick, she brought me to work with her; so, I grew up around the profession," he explains. "When I was 18, I joined an ambulance team in our small community in northwestern Ontario, Canada, as a volunteer and then went on to college to become an Emergency Medical Technician (EMT). However, I didn't like it when you would save one accident victim while another died and all you would hear about is the one who died, or taking someone to the emergency room and not knowing the outcome of the event. Nursing allows me to spend more time following a patient's progress."

As a male nurse, John admits to feeling stereotyped at times. "Actually," he reports, "it's similar to how women are stereotyped in other professions. In truth, a lot of nurses tell me they like to be on a shift with a male who can do more of the heavy lifting work. Also, in a general sense, male nurses may be viewed as being more feminine than masculine. In a female-dominated profession, society naturally considers nursing a 'motherly' type of career and not necessarily a profession. Nursing is a profession like any other and, as stereotypical as it sounds, until society experiences more males in nursing (along with other initiatives), it will be a while until they change their view despite the valiant effort of some professional nursing organizations. For example, a baccalaureate-prepared RN is educated extensively in pharmacology and carries a bachelor of science degree. As such, we are expected to perform many of the functions of a pharmacist along with dozens more activities, yet there remains a huge gap between the professions in terms of recognition and salary." Continuing, John informs us, "I experience uneasiness from some women, especially those in older generations, who expect men to be physicians, not nurses. A few people address me as 'doctor' when they see me for the first time. Some people even perceive male nurses as not being able to make it in medical school."

After graduating from nursing school, John returned to his small hometown community to practice at the local hospital. He gained extensive experience across a broad range of specialties, everything from OB to geriatrics. Becoming increasingly disillusioned by the Canadian socialistic medical climate, he and his wife packed their bags and headed for the United States in 1996. He knew fairly early in his career that he wanted to be in a leadership role, but to expand his experience, the two decided to become traveling nurses. He recounts, "The money was good; we could move every three months or so. We decided to visit all four corners of the country, following the seasons of the year. We worked in Maine and the state of Washington in the summer and Florida and New Mexico in the winter."

The idea of traveling internationally was appealing, and so he accepted a contract in Saudi Arabia where he was a nurse for the royal family and other V.I.P.'s at the King Faisal Specialist Hospital. "It rapidly became quite an experience because these people emerged from the desert only about 50 years ago," he reports. "They had billions of dollars thrust at them, so they could do whatever they wanted."

According to John, living in such a different culture was a challenge. "It was rather startling to observe and understand how differently woman were treated from men. In many ways, the culture appeared hypocritical; people often said one thing but did something else. For example, they say they segregate single women from men in order to protect them, when in reality, it appeared that women are viewed as being inferior. Religious police are there to enforce the rules of the Koran. Even my wife was hassled a few times.

"Also, you are sponsored to enter the country, but then they take possession of your passport, and you must go through a process to get it back in order to leave the country. They say they do this in case your family needs to contact you while away on a holiday, but in my opinion that was simply another method of exercising control."

While there, John worked his way from a staff nurse into a position as nursing supervisor and then manager in Ambulatory Care. After the birth of their first child, they decided to return to the United States where John accepted a managerial position in ambulatory services at the Rogue Valley Medical Center hospital in Medford, Oregon. Working toward his goal in administration, he asserts, "What I like best about management is being able to see the big picture and having the ability to influence a large number of people on my staff, which will eventually impact a greater number of patients and the care they receive.

| Skill Clusters | Transferable Skills |
|---|---|
| Strategist | Efficiency |
| Managerial Competence | Designing/Drawing |
| Technical Competence | Potential Problem-solving |
| Learning | Precision |
| Fellowship | Structuring |

John lists *strategist, managerial competence,* and *efficiency* as his top skills, critical to his job of supervising 75 direct reports in four areas of the hospital. "The four areas I manage are basically unique," he reports, "so I must build a support system to help me manage them. We operate with a coaching model, meaning that job descriptions are based upon accountabilities, and I meet with each employee several times a year so that expectations remain clear."

Not surprisingly, one of John's greatest frustrations is the inability to give as much one-on-one time to his staff as he would like, especially because he is fairly new in his job and is still orienting into the organization. He expresses having a great passion for his job. "One of my greatest joys is the ability to interact with a large number of people and make a difference in their lives and their work. I am able to sit back, listen, process information, see a pattern, and suggest alternatives and solutions," he states, evidence of his *potential problem-solving* ability. He thrives on responding spontaneously to different situations and solving problems. For John, variety is the "spice of life," indicative of his thoroughly enjoyable experience as a traveling nurse.

Because he basically embodies thinking and analytical orientations, our interview with John underscores the reality that there are many different ways to care for people, not just limited to the caring processes of feeling and emotion. John cares for others in a practical, here-and-now, expeditious manner. He also cares by *learning* from his staff and his patients, being open to new ideas and, whenever possible, not being restricted by onerous rules and regulations. He refuses to see all of the changes occurring today in health care as limiting his ability to care. Rather, they are opportunities to innovate. He believes firmly that there is always something that can be done differently without having to throw additional people and dollars at a problem.

John always views the glass as being neither half-full nor half-empty, but as something capable of being filled. As part of his personal development, he studies everything that he can find about models of constructive change. His personal motto is, "Let's get busy"; his motivation is to engage in the art of possibility as opposed to assuming limitations.

# WE'LL GET THERE!
Karen D. Beatty, MSN, RN, BSN
*Visiting nurse: African American PIPE queen*

As an African American nurse, Karen Beatty sometimes faces rejection from her patients. "We care just like anyone else and it saddens us, especially during these times of nurse shortages, to walk into a patient's room and on rare occasions to be turned away," she recounts. "My earlier hospital nursing experience included working in the Intensive Care Nursery (ICN). Today I work as a visiting nurse in Philadelphia. There are times I enter someone's home and can sense that I am not welcomed. They don't want the neighbors to see a black person coming into their home. Of course, I don't argue with them, but offer to schedule another nurse. But," she grins, "I'm an optimist and my motto is 'We'll get there!'" This attitude extends to her work with her clients.

Karen decided to enter nursing early in her life because of the excitement she felt around an aunt who was a nurse. When she had to make a paper doll in the first grade, Karen created a nurse with a brown face.

Karen attended an associate nursing program at a small Catholic college and was one of only two African Americans out of more than 100 graduating students. Coming to school from an urban area and being black, she found herself being stereotyped at first in the belief that she might steal from the other students. "But, I developed a number of good friends and really had many good experiences," she reports.

Karen's work as a visiting nurse spans over 10 years. In the beginning, she explains, her focus was in pediatrics and she worked in a very poor section of Philadelphia where 80% of her cases were related to drug abuse. She also worked with depressed mothers and people with a variety of mental illnesses. Her work coordinated with that of substance abuse specialists and social workers. "I had a caseload of about 125 clients and after about eight years, I was really getting burned out," she notes. Fortunately, funding was received to develop the Nurse-Family Partnership Program (NFP).

According to Karen, the NFP provides first-time, low-income mothers of any age with home visitation services from public health nurses. NFP nurses work intensively with these mothers to improve maternal, prenatal, and early childhood health and well-being with the expectation that this early intervention will help achieve long-term improvements in the lives of these at-risk families, states Karen. "The early intervention is effective because it focuses on developing therapeutic relationships with the family and is designed to improve five broad domains of family functioning: health (physical and mental), home and neighborhood environment, family and friend support, parental roles, and major life events (e.g., pregnancy planning, education, employment).

"My work environment now is a much healthier place for me," she believes. "Today, I serve only 25 clients. The NFP model protects the nurse because, with reflective supervision, you have a weekly consultation with your supervisor. Also, it serves as a collaborative program with several area universities and the Visiting Nurses Association.

"While the case load is manageable," she explains, "the situations often become quite intense. For example, I visit with mothers while they are pregnant and stay with them until their child reaches two years of age. I have clients attempting to get their GED and others who have been to college. Two of them must cope with mental disorders and another with unmanageable anger."

| Skill Clusters | Transferable Skills |
| --- | --- |
| Maximizing | Emotional Control |
| Creativity | Motor Coordination |
| Compassion | Responding to Pressure |
| Acceptance | Shape Discrimination |
| Relating | Potential Problem-solving |
| Flexibility | |
| Self-directing | |

Karen adapts to the intensity of her work by using her *maximizing* cluster of skills, maintaining an orientation toward seeing the best in people and helping them to act upon their strengths. It also relates to the "maintaining belief" process of caring, believing that there is meaning to be found in the situation and going the distance with a person. She maintains, "When we work with our clients in terms of vocational goals, we don't impose our own agendas. We go with whatever the client expresses as a heart's desire. I help people to believe that they can achieve their goals."

Continuing, Karen reports, "I have a client whose mother unfortunately died of a heart attack. Shortly thereafter she became pregnant and delivered a child. On top of that she has a seizure disorder. She is a very bright woman who graduated from high school. We helped her enter college and the first semester she received one 'A,' one 'F,' and three withdrawals. Her biggest problem is childcare and she had to stay at home because the welfare system fell through in terms of funding day care. However, thank God, she received one 'A' because that has motivated her to return to school."

This is one example of Karen's ability to seek out the "gold nuggets" in people. Then she uses her *creativity* and *compassion* skills to motivate them to move forward with their lives. Naturally sympathetic and caring, she receives tremendous gratification from seeing people do well. Once a single parent herself, she can relate to the challenges some of her clients face.

She relates, "I count it as a privilege to enter the lives of 25 different people, helping to mold them and to move them forward to better lives. One example of how I use my *creativity* in this respect entails how I use a manual called PIPE, or Partners in Parenting Education. The PIPE program teaches professionals to train parents in areas of communication, emotional regulation, and relationship building. Sometimes I'm called the 'pipe queen,' meaning that I can make a lesson out of virtually nothing," she says laughing. "I am blessed with the gift of communicating and helping people to understand and learn."

Nursing is a wonderful profession, Karen believes. "Not only do you give of yourself, but you have to be strong and open to change. For African Americans, it also means getting to know people and not judging all people on the basis of one individual's behavior."

Karen has learned the importance of caring for herself. Long a student of ballet and tap, she both performs and choreographs dance numbers. "I even choreographed a dance number for my boyfriend's family reunion," she says a little self-consciously.

It appears obvious that Karen finds great joy and purpose in her work. As an enabling educator and with her caring abilities to communicate and motivate, Karen makes her "We'll get there" attitude contagious. She is superbly positioned to perform the work of a visiting nurse. On the other hand, given the concerning shortages of nurses and nursing professors, her skills and abilities would make her an inspiring nurse educator.

# NURSING IN THE FOXHOLE

Amy Brown, BSN, RN

*Psychiatric nurse: Unconditional positive regard*

Amy Brown's work centers upon the art of communication. As she describes her work, every day is different and almost daily she must deal with a difficult situation. She laughs when she explains that someone once told her that she is the kind of person you want in a foxhole because she can communicate, lead people, and calm them down while exhibiting compassion.

Growing up, Amy found herself torn between teaching and nursing. However, when her father contracted cancer while she was still in college, she quickly had to adapt to being a caregiver. "I became intrigued not only from a medical perspective, but with what it was like to sit with a person through their treatment. At one point, my father told me that I would be a very good nurse. Also, my older sister is a nurse, so we have some family history in the profession."

As part of her nurse's training, Amy rotated through different specialties, including a six-week psychiatric rotation in a state hospital. "That experience still sticks with me," she recounts. "I've always had a curiosity about the mind, especially in neurological and psychiatric disciplines. I worked for a period of time in a neurological ICU and loved it."

For the past 10 years, Amy has worked in psychiatric nursing. She worked first as a nurse therapist and cofacilitated a number of outpatient groups. For the past three years, she has served as a program manager in a psychiatric unit in Boulder, Colorado.

Not surprisingly, Amy's key skill clusters include *communication* and *compassion*, important almost always in nursing but especially so in behavioral health. "No day is quite the same," she maintains, "and like ICUs, sometimes we must *respond to emergencies*. You must be *flexible*, because every patient in the unit is there for a different reason and presents their symptoms in a different manner."

As a psychiatric nurse, she must utilize all five processes of caring. She especially enjoys simply being with people, listening to them, and conveying understanding. She also spends much of her time enabling and *advising* her patients, teaching people how to care for themselves and how to work with their families. "People want to not only know what depression is all about but why they are depressed," she explains. "In that context, we attempt to view the entire tapestry of someone's life."

| Skill Clusters | Transferable Skills |
| --- | --- |
| Communication | Understanding/Tact |
| Flexibility | Conveying Emotions |
| Compassion | Advising |
| Leadership | Responding to Emergencies |
| Connectivity | Responding to Pressure |
| Self-directing | |
| Entrepreneurship | |

Amy's *leadership* and *entrepreneurship* skills came to the forefront about four years ago when she took a break from behavioral health care and opened a residential hospice care center. "I have a passion for this kind of work and may end up again in that arena before my career ends," she states. "Hospice can be psychiatric-oriented as well because much of it focuses upon mental preparation for death. I had to learn pain management, but much of what I learned in the behavioral sciences applied to hospice care. And, of course, often we must deal with a family's dynamics and complexities."

Because working in a psychiatric unit is not an easy arena, Amy is intentional in her efforts to care for her staff and assist them in caring for themselves. "First," she responds, "I am very visible to them. They appreciate the fact that I work alongside them in patient care. Also, I use a lot of humor," she grins. "Often psychiatric nurses become the targets of people's moods and anxieties, and humor becomes an important way to deflect such emotions. In addition, we conduct a lot of impromptu supervision meetings, and for the past three years, we have held retreats involving a lot of fun and play.

"On the medical side of health care, people often express their thanks for our service, whereas on the mental health side that is not always the case," she states reflecting. "That is why we need a lot of camaraderie and participation in positive group interaction, including nonnursing staff. Philosophically, I believe that the housekeepers are just as important to the team. They see and hear everything that we see and hear."

Amy also attempts to honor diversity in her team, not just in terms of ethnicity, but also in terms of personal style and temperament. "People's different personalities put together can create a wonderful tapestry for serving patients who are in different places. In a respectful manner, it becomes a matter of learning how to agree to disagree in the midst of this diversity. I engage in a lot of this practice," she relates. "I will say, 'I understand what you are saying, yet this is what we must do for the greater good.' It becomes a way of validating a person's experience without dismissing them."

Amy believes that caring entails giving unconditional respect and positive regard, both emotionally and physically. It necessitates being present in the moment and respecting the situation even if there is disagreement and requires self-discipline and consciousness. Giving positive regard means that your personal beliefs and judgments remain on the sideline.

As a psychiatric nurse, we asked Amy to reflect on the potential link between nursing and codependency. Codependence, as the term is used today, has various meanings. In general, it refers to how some past events starting in our childhood "unknowingly" affect some of our attitudes, behaviors, and feelings in the present, sometimes with destructive consequences. People are usually aware of codependency when it occurs. Signs of its presence include having low self-esteem, seeking validation through accomplishments, and feeling frustrated when they don't come.

"It often feels good to take care of other people, but you can't enter the profession expecting that it will be the outcome," Amy says emphatically. "Probably no career exists that will completely fulfill one's need to be appreciated and esteemed by others. We are continually addressing and facing those personal needs. I happen to believe that a desire to serve and to care resides as a core belief for the majority of people. When I worked in hospice, I viewed it as a complete privilege to be in someone's home or room as they were dying. Even in psychiatric work, it becomes a privilege to be in a space with someone when they are so scared and they are exhibiting symptoms such as paranoia or hallucinations. In any case, we need to keep balance. One does not need to be of service 24 hours a day. When I interview people for a position, I often recommend a half-time job in the psychiatric unit coupled with half-time work in another unit. Also, during performance reviews, I inform my people that when they stop choosing to do this kind of work and yet feel they cannot leave it, they need to consider looking for another job. In reality, I want to know when an employee of mine decides to look for another job because I want to help them find it. It would solve a lot of the current problems in health care if this attitude were more universally adopted by managers. We need to focus on a supportive environment for employees and work on retention of good nurses in our hospitals rather than just for our units or departments."

Not surprising, one of Amy's heroes is Mother Teresa. "I've been interested in her for years," she reports. "If what I read about her is true, my admiration stems from her devotion to service in an almost completely nonattached manner. She apparently enjoyed her commitment to making the world a better place. She didn't expect anything in return. I believe that when we can give without expecting a return, then, if and when it is returned to us, we can more readily appreciate it."

Amy remains optimistic about the future of health care, but believes that some cultural changes need to be made. "We need to strengthen the sense of enjoyment in the profession," she maintains. "Nurses go into health care because they want to be with people. I've never heard anyone say they entered nursing for money, for power, or for factors you often see in other areas of work," proclaims Amy. "People enter nursing to learn and practice the art of caring; so we must strengthen this model and provide innovative benefits, perhaps by offering sabbaticals, increased education, and self-care opportunities or whatever else it may take to help nurses renew a commitment to their careers. I also strongly believe in the importance of nurturing nurses throughout their careers. We must be caregivers of ourselves and our colleagues to maintain a healthy and positive caregiver role in our careers."

At the end of her life, Amy would be pleased if someone honored her commitment to serving people and to being a compassionate, enjoyable person in her relationships with her colleagues and patients. She asserts, "I would like my life of service to be commemorated. I would like it said that I enjoyed doing it and had fun in the process! And all in all, nursing has been a fulfilling and rewarding career path for me."

# HAVE A PLAN

Bettina Pangan, BSN, RN

*Clinical analyst seeing both sides of care*

For someone not intending to become a nurse, Tina Pangan is passionate about nursing. "I come from a family of educators. My mother is a retired librarian/ teacher. I am the renegade in the family!" Tina says laughing. "My first idea was to become a librarian, but my mother talked me out of that. I am really too noisy to be a librarian," she grins. "Everyone at work tells me to quiet down. My friends were going into nursing, so I thought I would try it, although I really didn't like science." It wasn't until the last two years of nursing school that nursing became her passion. "I loved cardiology," she explains. "You could actually see and hear what was happening to the heart of a patient, and I loved the interaction with people. Not only could I give part of myself, but I got so much in return back from my patients; that's when the passion for the profession began to build."

Tina's love of nursing grew deeper as her education and nursing experiences progressed. Even what appeared to be a career setback further affirmed her decision. "At one point, I thought I might like to become a computer programmer. But, you had to score pretty high on the math exam to get into the program and I didn't." Although disappointing at the time, she later viewed it as a sign to keep pursuing a nursing degree. "Of course, today, I am glad that I didn't go into that field. I would not have been happy. My friends laugh at me because I must always have a plan. If one thing doesn't work out, I almost always have a contingency plan. I am a very practical person!"

An Asian American with Spanish great-grandparents, Tina emigrated from the Philippines to the United States as a teenager. She finished high school in New Mexico and, after marrying in her sophomore year of college, she moved to California where she obtained an associates degree in nursing. Because Tina found it difficult as a new nursing graduate living in a new community to find a job in acute care, she accepted a position as an RN Charge Nurse in a 99-bed long-term-care facility. This decision profoundly affected her future career path. "I found my job rewarding and one that really made me feel like I made a difference. However, I was young and, after three years, I thought that I was losing the wonderful clinical skills I had mastered in my

ADN program. So, I moved to an acute care Catholic hospital, but still tried to work part-time in long-term care because the seniors made an impact in my life."

Returning to Albuquerque, she finished her BSN and worked in a cardiac step-down unit at Presbyterian Hospital. Subsequent positions included working in the quality department where she was involved in projects building clinical paths and performance improvement initiatives. She later worked in the health plan as a community nurse case manager for the managed care senior and commercial members, a position she thoroughly enjoyed.

Today, she is a clinical analyst conducting descriptive studies and working with a team to develop interventions for patient populations. "When I left case management, I didn't realize just how much I would miss the patient contact and the feeling that I am here for a purpose," she says. Tina's love of working with seniors led her to enroll in a master's program to obtain a degree as a family nurse practitioner. "Caring for seniors is my passion," she affirms. "My departed grandmother has been my inspiration. When I look back at my 18-year nursing career, I find that the time I spent with older people (regardless of setting) as being the most rewarding." When she completes her degree, she plans to resume working with maturing adults. "I've stopped calling them seniors," she says. "They have so much wisdom, and I have so much to learn from their stories. I am grateful for my time with them. Also, I think my experience working on the health plan side of medicine will make me a better nurse."

Part of her plan includes entering the U.S. Public Health Commissioned Corps with her husband, also a family nurse practitioner. "The Corps is one of the uniformed services that many people don't know about," she reports. But for Tina, that may not work out because of the upper age limit for obtaining a commission. "I will be just under it when I finish my degree; so, we'll see. But," she grins, "I have my alternative plan. I can always continue nursing at Presbyterian; it really is an excellent place to work. Nurses are genuinely empowered through the nursing councils." In the future, teaching may be on her agenda should she get her PhD.

| Skill Clusters | Transferable Skills |
| --- | --- |
| Accountability | Dependability |
| Achievement-oriented | Drive/Tenacity |
| Strategist | Performing |
| Learning | Analyzing |
| Analytical | Planning |
| Self-directing | |
| Artistic | |

Tina especially uses key skill clusters of *accountability* and *strategist* to build firm foundations for her life and work. "Patient care is very purposeful and certainly a good nurse must be competent and accountable," she underscores. "I also enjoy mentoring people. In fact, when I worked on the floor, I was a preceptor and coached the newer nurses. Of course, patient education is an important function of a nurse practitioner."

Tina loves to *learn* and can get bored quite easily, so it is understandable why she is working on a master's degree and may follow it with a doctorate. She enjoys reading her textbooks. For her, learning becomes a form of self-care, as well as the enjoyment she receives from using her *analytical* skills to apply the learning in creative ways. Her *drive/tenacity* is used to increase her competence, allowing her to acquire new information and master new concepts. She loves to raise questions and probably would not thrive in a "do what you are told" type of environment. Rather, she uses her intuition to anticipate needs and to determine what to do about them.

Dorothea Orem's self-care model serves as the foundation for her nursing practice. "The basic premise is that humans are self-care agents," she relates, "and when they can no longer take care of themselves, that is when nursing care takes over at various levels." The theory postulates three types of nursing systems:

- *Wholly compensatory* systems are required for individuals unable to do anything for themselves, controlling and monitoring their environment and processing information;
- *Partially compensatory* systems are designed for individuals who are unable to perform some (but not all) self-care activities;
- *Supportive-educative (developmental)* systems are necessary for persons who need to learn to perform self-care measures and need assistance to do so.

This theory gives the patient the opportunity to retain or to regain some type of control during or after a health episode and is based upon the patient's perception, not that of the caregiver.

Tina explains that three tenets guide her. The first involves education. "I believe that education is important and coming from a family of educators, education is obviously a family creed. Second, I believe in being true to one's self (even if it means going against the grain), and the third is rising above adversity. I don't believe in wallowing in a pool of sorrow or playing victim. Rise above it; don't complain (well, maybe sometimes it is necessary to be heard) and do something about it!"

Tina underscores the importance of nurses taking care of themselves in order to care for others. "Nurses need to recognize when they are getting to a burnout phase and plan breaks," she says. "Then, decide what steps you are going to take in order to do something about it." Tina reports taking care of herself by laughing a lot and utilizing reflection and prayer. "I love learning, and I like to reflect on things and find joy in little things. I think it's important to be grateful for what you have. There is a saying, 'Happiness is not getting what you want, but being grateful for what you have.' I would add, have a goal because it may not happen! In fact, if you can't find anything to be grateful about in your current situation, then it is time to move on."

Tina also emphasizes the importance of working in an environment where employers and managers care about people. "I believe managers have to be sincere in their efforts to know their staff; that builds trust. People have to be validated for what they achieve as a person and for what they do professionally.

"Nursing is a great profession because it connects you to people," Tina says enthusiastically. "Nursing is really both art and science. People can learn the skills, the technical proficiencies, but unless they have the passion for caring, they will burn out. I hope other people who have emigrated understand that it's possible to come to this country, receive an education, and do whatever they want. Just look at me! I hope my example inspires others who are considering nursing as a career."

# SOCIAL NURSE-A-WORKER

Marianne Davis, RN

*Legendary strategist: Piloting people through the healthcare maze*

Marianne Davis often introduces herself as a "social nurse-a-worker" because she believes the coined term best represents her work, a combination of her two careers. Sometimes when she speaks to groups, she is introduced as a "living legend." She seems surprised at the designation. For her, life simply has been a succession of opportunities, and in some ways she has forged her own journey's path.

Marianne's original career goal was to become a nurse when she entered Linfield College in Oregon. However, the program's required summer work and five years of study were obstacles at that time in her life. Needing to finance her own education, she chose an alternative career in social work.

After graduation, she worked as a social services case manager until her first child was born. Re-entering the workforce when her children reached school age, she found a position as a paraprofessional teacher in the Seattle school system, which gave her greater flexibility. Working in a high school biology department rekindled an interest in nursing. She recalls, "So, when a school financing levy failed to pass at the polls and I lost my job, I took my retirement funds and used them to finance my nursing education. By this time, two-year programs were available at the community colleges." She discovered that her teaching experience was invaluable in her later work.

After graduation, she took a hospital nursing job with Good Samaritan Hospital in Puyallup (pronounced Pew-al-up), Washington. She remained in that capacity for five years until the hospital applied for a Robert Wood Johnson grant, an initiative designed to demonstrate what hospitals could do in the arena of long-term care. When the hospital received the grant, Marianne applied for the new position because she saw it as an opportunity to integrate her social work, teaching, and nursing skills.

She relates, "After being a hospital nurse, it felt wonderful to go out to people's homes. In the hospital, shifts changed every eight hours. Doctors gave us orders and there were very strict procedures to adhere to. On the other hand, in the home it was the spouse or other family members who were the caregivers. Some of the caring duties were heavy and time-consuming, but very loving and dedicated, often performed with mixed emotions. I discovered that caregivers did not always follow the doctor's instructions. Noncompliance is a rather negative term, but often there were some very valid reasons why people could not do what the doctor prescribed.

"For example," she continues, "a doctor prescribed blood pressure medication that didn't seem to be working. The doctor kept increasing the dosage until finally the daughter discovered that her father wasn't taking the medication because he could not open the bottle. She opened it for him, but by this time the dosage was so high the man fell and broke his hip. So often physicians don't understand the stresses involved in home care.

"Through training, I gradually began to realize that dementia patients are not being deliberately difficult and to see that there were a variety of strategies available that might make things easier. For example, a daughter of a patient told me, 'I don't know what we are going to do with mother. She keeps urinating in a can and putting it under her bed.' I asked her to think back to earlier times; that is what you did on the farm when there was no inside bathroom. Her mother was back there in time. 'Oh,' said the daughter. This knowledge made it possible for the family to better understand her and to be kinder."

Marianne reports that the essential task in dealing with people with dementia is to relate to them at the feeling level and not with logic or facts. She tells a wonderful story, though not experienced personally, about a man named Jim living with dementia in a nursing home. He continually asked, "What time does the train leave for Boise [Idaho]? I need to go home to Boise." The nurses all tried to reason with him, stating that he was in a nursing home and that there was no train to Boise. The man became angry and threw things. Finally, a housekeeper who didn't know that you were supposed to focus upon reality, said, "Jim, there is no train coming today, but you can stay at our hotel." She was responding to the underlying feeling of being disoriented and lost. Jim continued asking when the train was coming, but he seemed satisfied with the answer.

Marianne laughs, "I always felt that I couldn't believe they were paying me to do this work. This was especially true when I went to visit homes in the South Puget Sound area, driving across the Tacoma Narrows Bridge with its view of Mt. Rainier. Not only was the driving environment pleasant, but also the people I served were always so grateful. Of course, there were difficult situations, but most people were very thankful for the resources I brought to them. When we conducted surveys about our service, the most common comments reflected gratitude for knowing that someone was available to call upon."

Marianne talks about how she brings her faith system into her nursing. She reports, "There have been some times when I have been asked to pray with a patient. Of course, in a hospital setting, we need to be somewhat more careful. Often, without the use of words, you can sense a spirit-to-spirit type of relationship, or, if you wish, soul-to-soul. I think of soul as the essence of a person, what they *are* apart from what they *do* in life. As a nurse, sometimes it's easy to misplace this distinction.

"For example, I remember visiting a woman who was to undergo gall bladder surgery. She was semi-sleeping when I approached her, hair messed up, drooling at the mouth, and wearing one of those ugly gowns that hospitals dispense to patients. However, later I saw a picture that her family brought to the hospital; it revealed a well-groomed, professional-looking woman. I said to myself that I needed to remember that people have diverse lives; this woman wasn't simply a gall bladder in Room 182, but a person."

Marianne also affirms the relationship between soul enhancement and storytelling. She speaks about an elderly blind woman who came to the hospital from a nursing home. Marianne recalls, "I began to bathe her, which is a perfect time to talk to people. I asked her what she had done for a living when she was younger. She spoke at great length about being a teacher in a one-room schoolhouse in Oregon. She received $60 per month and the free use of a horse. The school board did not allow any dances to be held in the building. Nevertheless, one time she organized a dance, primarily because the kids had very little to do with their leisure time. She heard a knock on the door and thought it must be a school board member, so she jumped out the window. Then, as I was finishing up with her bath and replacing the bed linen, suddenly, she said to everyone in the room, 'Everyone take out a piece of clean, white paper for the spelling test.' She became so caught up in her reminiscing, that she was imaginatively back in the classroom."

Since that experience, Marianne has read considerable material about the value of reminiscing. Positive or negative, people re-experience the emotions associated with an event. In his book *Dancing Healers*[7] (1989), Carl Hammerschlag, MD, informs us that saying the words "Remember when . . ." places the audience in an altered state of consciousness—the very act of remembering often makes us spellbound. This is especially true for people with dementia who often have access to long-term as opposed to recent memory.

Entering this field became a huge challenge for Marianne, she remembers. At the time, she knew nothing about dementia, so it was quite a learning experience. Over the years, Marianne has devoted much of her energies to this area and to aging in general. Although her career has been varied, she describes her work over the past 15 years as being most satisfying. During that period, until her retirement (we use the word guardedly because she remains very active in health care), she served as a family outreach nurse. Knowing that she didn't have to worry about performing procedures that could be life threatening, she was able to apply her broad knowledge to a variety of healthcare issues.

As an example, she reports, "I worked with one daughter who was beside herself over the condition of her mother. When I got to the house for the first time, I discovered that the mother refused to visit a doctor. She hadn't seen one for about 50 years, since her son was born. She had legs dripping with pus, but the daughter could not get her to go to the hospital. So, I racked my brain attempting to arrive at a strategy," Marianne remembers. "First, I played upon her love for her daughter and the feeling of guilt about the frustration she was causing. Then, I turned to hope by explaining that I had seen worse infections and this could be taken care of. She finally consented to go to the emergency room!"

This incident serves as an excellent example of one of Marianne's key skill clusters, namely *strategist*. She is a friendly persuader who will use any strategy that may work for gaining a positive outcome with a patient. In fact, the woman with infected legs eventually left the hospital to enter a nursing home. Marianne received a lovely letter from the daughter informing her that her mother finally returned to her home.

| Skill Clusters | Transferable Skills |
| --- | --- |
| Analytical | Analyzing |
| Learning | Understanding/Tact |
| Compassion | Serving |
| Acceptance | Training |
| Strategist | Reading |
| Maximizing | |
| Service/Dedication | |

Marianne also enjoys using her *analytical* skills. For example, her nursing education did not provide her with any training on setting up traction. She states, "I would analyze information in manuals, then follow through with an actual patient. In more than one occasion, I came to realize that the book was wrong. So, it pays to question," she declares emphatically.

As mentioned earlier, although officially retired, Marianne remains actively interested in health care. She enrolled in a few courses on parish nursing and is currently exploring this field as an avocation. A Methodist, Marianne established a health ministry group promoting physical, emotional, and spiritual health through a variety of projects, such as giving blood pressure checks, presenting classes on aging, and holding health fairs. One project having the greatest impact is a care team ministry. Most team members are assigned to one or two senior citizens, but could easily take on more short-term assignments, she believes. She sees much room for growth in the group's work by providing more support to the paid pastoral staff.

Marianne is concerned with care of those who are aging. "In general, people are lumped together in one age group of '65 and older,'" she complains. Yet, she says, there is a great disparity between those who have just retired and people who are in their 80s or older. As she argues, "This represents just one reason why we need to identify more transitional periods for people and to develop appropriate rituals to assist passage through them. We need a ritual for someone who turns 65 and leaves a paid, 40-hour-a-week job. And certainly, we need a ritual for those who must leave home and move into some form of assisted living. That there are no such rituals available, even in organized religion, bears unfortunate witness to the denial of the aging process and to stereotyping."

# PASSIONATE TENACITY

Naomi Mason, BSN, RN, PHN
*Native American Shoshone obstacle remover*

If there is one word that describes Naomi Mason, it is tenacious. As a Shoshone Indian, she was born and raised in an isolated area on the Death Valley Indian Reservation straddling the Idaho/Nevada border. The Shoshone nation is perhaps best known for the story of Sacagawea, the Native American woman who traveled westward with the Lewis and Clark expedition.

Early on, Naomi states, there were no gravel roads and no electricity. And yet, she believes that it was a wonderful life filled with many changes. Native Americans are always in transition and have been since Caucasian people came to the American continent, she reminds us. At the age of 18, her father journeyed to the Carlisle Indian School in Pennsylvania to study, and he knew the famous athlete Jim Thorpe. He constantly amazed the family with his interest in politics and his love of operatic singing.

"On the other hand," she states, "My mother was a victim of circumstances. She was very brilliant and taught herself how to read and write. She continually read books and almost everything she could put her hands on. However, both my parents experienced constant fear from living in a dominant white society and, of course, so did I. My mother told me stories about the times when Indian women reached puberty. The ritual attached to this event was for the woman to enter a small tent for a period of time to contemplate and meditate on this transition into adulthood. It was a very sacred event, but the white soldiers sometimes came around, roping the woman and dragging her away to be raped. There was little the men of the tribe could do because there was always a gun at their heads."

Naomi grew up in an environment where she received many conflicting messages. She was a Shoshone Indian, yet her parents were converted Presbyterians, and the family attended church each Sunday. She reports, "I had one foot in Western culture, yet my aunt was a medicine woman who healed with herbs. This is one reason why I chose nursing as a profession. In addition, I am an innately curious person," she confesses. "We raised a lot of chickens and when one of them died prematurely, I would open it up and try to find the cause!"

One of Naomi's daughters, Francesca (Fran), was present during the interview. "One of the traits I most admire in my mother is her intelligence," she says. "I admire her multidimensional experience and expertise. She remains such a relevant resource for all of her children. I have many reasons to respect her simply as a woman and as a healer. But above all, my sisters and I have said that, with our mother, we don't have any excuses. We can't say, 'Oh, I can't do that because . . .' Any excuse must be thrown out the window. At the very least, for us, she is a pioneer! Her inspiration undoubtedly impacted two of my sisters. One sister is the director of the Women's Health Specialists clinic in Redding, California, working with disadvantaged women. My other sister just received her doctorate in law."

Chuckling, Fran recalls that her mother was never *not* a nurse, even before becoming an RN. "I remember when my brother walked straight into the branch of a tree, a twig went directly into his eye. At the time, Mom was a housewife, but came out, clipped the twig, holding the eye open. When the doctor dilated his eye, the twig came out without injury. Even today, she continues to help our rather large family whenever problems or disabilities develop."

Naomi recounts the difficultly she experienced living in a dominant white society and being accepted as a Native American. "You were either this or that, Caucasian or Indian; you couldn't just be a human, holographic being," she remembers. Yet, according to Naomi, everyone who is bicultural is both. If not, she believes people end up denying part of themselves.

Naomi went to boarding school in Riverside, California. However, she felt herself to be a misfit because of the fear inherited from her parents related to how white people treated Native Americans. So, after only one year, she returned home, desiring only to remain on the reservation. Her parents, however, wanted more for her and not knowing what to do, finally turned to their Presbyterian pastor. He immediately located a home for her in Berkeley, California, where she worked as a housekeeper and babysitter in exchange for attending high school.

Again, Naomi experienced tremendous cultural shock. She turned down a scholarship to attend nursing school mainly because she was taught not to ask for "handouts." She was raised to earn her own way. So she worked as a housemaid for a period of time, saved her money, and then paid her own way for one and a half years before falling in love and leaving nursing school to get married. After giving birth to seven children and then divorcing, she returned to school in 1968.

After graduation, Naomi began working in an Intensive Care Unit. She states, "I especially enjoy working on a one-to-one basis where I am able to make appropriate decisions. But eventually, I returned home thinking that the reservation might be a better place to raise my last two children. I received additional education in Indian health services. It became ideal for me because it was again mostly one-on-one. I loved it because I was out in the field and in people's homes, covering seven tribes over a wide area. My work involved making autonomous decisions. I was accepted because I am one of them and they have my deepest respect. Also, these people experience a deep connection to soul. It's interesting, because we don't have a word for spirit; the only word we have is *mukua*, the word for soul. Spirit is a non-Indian word, yet for us, everything is sacred."

Today, Naomi teaches a parenting course for first-time offenders through the University of Nevada. Though the program is actually for young people, the parents must participate. The course helps people communicate with each other. She limits her teaching to just four hours each week because, as she says, "I'm just too busy to invest more of myself in this project. I'm involved in tribal politics and serve on the enrollment committee; not everyone qualifies to be a tribal member. I also have three aging sisters who need my help. They are all older and I believe I have a responsibility to them.

"I think my life has been an interesting journey and I am looking forward to the next chapter," she muses. "I plan to teach a class for certified nurses' aids. I want to appeal to many of the younger people to consider nursing as a profession. At the moment, I am asking for guidance to make certain that I follow the right path," she smiles.

It comes as no surprise that one of Naomi's key skill clusters is *self-directing*, being guided by an inner compass. She reports that she has always been blunt, even in the midst of early childhood fears. It becomes a good technique for her, because it doesn't allow for self-deception. Also, especially in her earlier days, becoming a nurse as a Native American meant overcoming considerable adversity. For Naomi, it surfaces in her transferable skill of *drive/tenacity*, helping her to overcome some of the obstacles involved in her education. For example, studying English represented quite a chore because it was not her first and dominant language.

| Skill Clusters | Transferable Skills |
|---|---|
| Learning | Using facts |
| Compassion | Flexibility |
| Flexibility | Understanding/Tact |
| Self-directing | Drive/Tenacity |
| Achievement | Decision-making |
| Accountability | |
| Acceptance | |

Naomi identifies *flexibility* as one of her most important abilities, which she has utilized throughout her life. She proclaims, "It is the reason that I was able to leave home and enter school in a different state in spite of the cultural shock. Because I grew up in two cultures, I had to be flexible. In addition, I worked with some Indian people who were extremely destitute. I had to set up a treatment plan that was within a person's reality. If I couldn't handle a situation, I could always call back to a doctor, but normally I was very autonomous."

Naomi's flexibility even shows up in her passion for *learning*. Like her mother, she is a fervent reader. She reads everything, going on "reading binges," devouring diverse subjects, everything from World War II to her Native American heritage.

Another one of Naomi's key skill clusters is *compassion*. When asked to describe what it meant, she responded, "Compassion embraces the enthusiasm of how I throw myself into work. It's all-consuming, which leads to how I care for others. I use compassion in all of the processes of caring. I also believe in the importance of compassionate touching. I learned this from both my mother and father, as well as from my Indian culture. We are a very tactile people. During some rituals, there is so much hugging that you can become exhausted by it. However, there exists a certain mindset in the Shoshone culture, and it probably exists in other Indian traditions as well, that if you perform therapeutic touching, you must be in a certain healthy place yourself. It is not an applied technique that anyone can use regardless of his or her circumstance."

Naomi believes one of the more passionate aspects of making a difference as a nurse is helping people to die in peace. Always present to listen, she affirms, "The Shoshones embrace the aging process, although it is sometimes quite difficult for others in the Western culture to do so. I believe that if it is a good death, that is, if there is no unfinished business or unforgiven relationships involved, then the soul leaves the body in great peace and goes wherever the soul goes. Also, the latest assumption, somewhat supported by science, is that some consciousness continues after death. This is why the ancient Indians believed that everything spoke—the animals, the hills, the rocks all talked and did so even before there were people on earth."

# CARING WITH A DISCERNING EYE
### Sandi Harding, MA, RN
*Parish nurse: Hugs and blessings*

Listening to Sandi Harding speak about her passion for parish nursing, it seems clear that she embodies caring through a discerning eye. Discernment involves standing beside a person in such a way as to determine the true situation and the actual need without projecting one's own agenda upon that person. It includes the gift of having a "spiritual eye" for cutting through facades and confusion to get to the heart of an issue.

For Sandi, caring flows naturally from being connected with soul. "Soul reflects our inner being, partly our character and partly our beliefs, a sense of who we are and what we are becoming. Soul is the way I would recognize you as a person if I could not see you," she avows.

Interestingly, she addresses human caring in a similar manner. It involves viewing another person as a unique individual and putting aside one's own agenda, values, and preoccupations. She suggests an image of "coming beside another person," knowing that we cannot enter the skin of that person to know completely her or his experiences, thoughts, and feelings. As such, caring entails taking the time to learn about a person without passing judgment, looking into someone's eyes and seeing what is needed. She explains, "It includes being transparent to another person, allowing another individual to feel safe enough to reveal parts of themselves and to share their stories. When we do this, then the time spent together is not a superficial meeting. This is not always an easy thing to do," she confesses.

In his book *Caring*[8] (1981), Morton Kelsey supports this viewpoint. "We are not exhausted by our rational consciousness. Our dreams, mistakes, fantasies, intuitions and mental quirks all remind us that there is something within us more than our rational, conscious mind and our sense experience."

A recent patient herself, Sandi recalls, "One evening a nurse came into my room and repositioned me with pillows behind my back and legs. I remembered the hundreds of times I did that with my patients, but being on the receiving side allowed me to experience this simple act of caring. It's just an undemanding extra step that communicates that a person is a real human and not just a medical case. But, unfortunately, today many nurses are being stretched so thin that often little or no time is available to take that extra, small step."

Sandi believes that touch plays a vital role in caring, be it a hand on the shoulder or an arm around the body. "As an Anglican," she informs us, "we pass the 'peace of the Lord' at church, embracing and hugging. Some people tell me that they had to come to church that day just for my hugs. I knew a minister who taught me how to hug, almost as an art form."

Even as a little girl, Sandi knew that nursing would be her passion. "Looking back upon it," she reflects, "sometimes I wondered whether this was my choice because career options for women were rather limited to nursing, teaching, or becoming a stay-at-home mom. But I can remember my grandmother telling me that I would be a terrific nurse. Also, my very favorite book was Nancy Nurse, and I went through a number of doctor's kits as a child," she laughs. "I had a life-size baby doll and pretended it was injured so I could bandage it; so there was something inside of me calling me to this profession."

Unfortunately, she says, there were many years when she couldn't wait to leave her career. Divorcing in the early 1980s was a life-changing event. She had married at the age of 19 and 11 years later, was raising three children alone. "I began to reassess why I entered nursing in the first place," she remembers. "It was the compassion and care giving, not the emergencies and the life-saving aspects of it." So, she went back to school and obtained a bachelor's degree in counseling. However, a problem developed with her oldest son, which prevented her from continuing toward a requisite master's degree.

At about the same time, Sandi accepted a management position that allowed her to work in an oncology unit Monday through Friday. She found that she was able to utilize her counseling skills on an almost daily basis with the patients, family, and staff alike. Smiling, she says, "At the same time, I developed a singles ministry at my church that included a program helping people transition through divorce. To this day, I continue to speak nationally on single parenting and divorce recovery."

As Sandi struggled with the existential question of "Why am I here?" she recalls thinking about the possibility of attending seminary and pursuing ministry full-time. "Then, when I first heard about the concept of parish ministry, that was it," she exclaimed. "I'll never forget the beautiful, sunny day, sitting in a swimming pool with a good friend of mine in Pittsburgh. Our hospital just merged with another one. We were both in middle management positions and pondering the direction of our careers when the subject of parish nursing came up. And I said with great conviction, 'That's it!' At the same time," she grins, "I had no clue as to what it meant to be a parish nurse! A friend conducted some research on the Internet and found out about a conference on parish nursing in Chicago, which I attended."

At the same time, Sandi was working toward a master's degree in a new leadership program at Duquesne University. She used the opportunity to focus all of her research papers upon parish nursing as she networked throughout the country. When she was offered a position in Atlanta, she immediately sold her home of 18 years and moved, leaving her son, daughter-in-law, and three grandchildren behind. "This was a step out in faith on my own! Everything I had worked for over the years came together," she smiles. "Throughout my life, all of those other little steps were leading me in this direction. It was a wonderful feeling. Earlier, I reflected upon what else I could do besides nursing. Before becoming a manager, I worked in the Intensive Care Unit (ICU). Always, my focus was less upon the adrenalin rush of urgent care and more on the compassionate side of nursing—being with the patients emotionally and guiding their families."

| Skill Clusters | Transferable Skills |
|---|---|
| Relating | Serving |
| Compassion | Understanding/Tact |
| Service/Dedication | Dependability |
| Communication | Cooperating |
| Self-directing | Explaining |
| Flexibility | |
| Stability/Security | |

Sandi distinguishes between healing and curing. So often in the medical profession we go for the physical cure. However, a person can experience healing emotionally and become whole without the physical body becoming cured of a disease or ailment.

Sandi utilizes many of her key satisfying skills during counseling sessions with people, especially with respect to issues of loss. "For example," she relates, "I had a woman brought to me who had suddenly experienced an anxiety attack while attending a meeting at church. I had her do some breathing exercises as a way of regaining control of her emotions. Then, I sought to understand what had triggered the attack. She was a widow in her 70s who had just started to date again and was getting into bad relationships. Both the woman's husband and her mother were alcoholics, but she had never dealt with these issues or attended an Al-Anon group. I approached her using my *relating* skills in a nonjudgmental manner and was able to make an appropriate referral."

Sandi also uses her ability to express *understanding/tact* in a manner that does not cross the boundary lines leading to codependence. She can be available and be present when needed without taking on too much responsibility for the outcome, but finding the appropriate resources for a given situation. Sharing another story, she tells of working with a family where the husband faced a terminal illness. She introduced the family to the services of hospice. Again, she speaks of caring as it relates to coming beside another person. Once she discerns the person's needs, she then uses the process of *enabling*, providing information and assisting him or her in making appropriate decisions. Sandi also takes pride in her transferable skill of *dependability*.

Sandi reminds us that the parish nursing model generally excludes clinical treatment of acute physical illnesses, although people may need to deal with the grief associated with such problems. Many of the individuals she sees do have chronic problems, such as high blood pressure or diabetes. She provides ongoing blood pressure monitoring and offers education related to the person's specific problem. She also offers educational materials for those who may have received a new diagnosis.

Not everyone she sees is a patient. For example, she ministered to a man who had come because his fairly young wife had just been diagnosed with a severe liver disease. He wanted her to refer him to other people who suffered from the same problem. "I continued to be a resource to him and met him at a few of the healing services that our congregation holds," she states quietly. "The woman passed away a few months after the diagnosis. The husband contacted me some time later and confessed that her loss was more difficult then he could have imagined. He wondered why the hurt remained so intense. I was able to connect him with a grief support group. Later, I learned that he had become a small group facilitator himself and was mentoring some of the men in it. Today, he vibrates with life."

While not focusing much time and energy upon clinical issues, Sandi does coordinate screening events for prostate cancer, skin cancer, osteoporosis, and the like. "I'm not big on health fairs, but I am more interested in education based upon one topic at a time, or one-on-one services," she reports. In addition, she joins us in observing a need for nurse advocates, who can explain a patient's options. "Absolutely, advocacy is included in my service, and I am able to do this on a more personal and oftentimes spiritual level," she affirms.

As part of her own self-caring strategies, Sandi allows herself to have "down days." Every day does not have to be filled with going somewhere and doing something. It calls to mind the admonition, "Don't just do something; stand there!" "For me," she states, "it may consist of sitting outside in the sunshine and reading a book. Or, I enjoy being with good friends, seeing a movie, or having enjoyable conversations over dinner." Sandi made a conscious decision to separate her place of work from her place of worship. Of course, she has many friends in the Methodist congregation where she works, but her support system and primary relationships are found in the Anglican Church she attends.

"I also have four grandchildren who refresh me when I am in their presence," she says proudly. "There is something about the smell of a newborn baby that brings delight to my senses. Then too, I find great peace when I'm in the presence of water. It can be a small stream or a huge ocean, although now living in Atlanta, it becomes harder to find such a place of solitude for self-care and reflection.

"Some people equate self-care with selfishness. When I went through my divorce, I became quite concerned about how I was going to care for three children by myself. However, I was counseled to take care of and heal myself first." She believes this is very important advice for anyone's self-care.

Because Sandi took this advice to heart and continues to do so, she seldom—if ever—experiences *compassion fatigue*, a phrase that sometimes replaces the more familiar term "burnout." The term refers to a physical, emotional, and spiritual fatigue or exhaustion that can consume a person and lead to a decline in his or her ability to experience joy or to feel and care for others. For Sandi, it's just the opposite. She becomes energized by numerous, meaningful relationships, from which flows her ability to compassionately care with a discerning eye.

# Part II
## Strategies for Organizational and Individual Caring

*Sometimes I wonder if anyone sees me,*
  *The skilled professional.*
   *The committed humanitarian.*
  *The caring human being.*
  *The solitary provider.*
  *The weary worker.*
*Sometimes I feel*
*Like an expendable commodity.*
  *Like an unwelcome intruder.*
  *Like a necessary inconvenience.*
  *Like an official afterthought.*
  *Like a worn out shoe.*
*Most of the time*
    *I work.*
    *I give.*
    *I care.*
    *I reflect.*
    *I love.*
  *And I don't have time to ponder the*
*"sometimes."*

—Kathy Sitzman, RN, Assistant Nursing Professor,
Weber State University, Ogden, Utah
and home healthcare nurse
(Printed with permission)

# Part IV

## Strategies for Organizational and Individual Caring

# Creating Healthy,
# Caring Organizational
# Culture—Strategies
# and Resources

Creating caring environments in which nurses can thrive is not a simple task. It requires commitment, a willingness to change, and a view to the possible. In the course of writing this book, we talked with a number of people from different areas of the country and in different healthcare settings about how organizations can be intentional in creating an environment that is healthy and caring for both patients and staff. Undoubtedly, the resources and strategies we share in this chapter do not represent all the innovative activities that are happening around the country. However, we believe that these are in some measure representative of best practices. We invite our readers to consider these strategies and to use them as a springboard in your own settings.

Arguably, having the support and commitment of the leadership in creating a culture that encourages the development and nurturing of a caring environment is critical. We also strongly believe that seeds for such development can be planted one individual and one unit at a time. As you will see, the Healing Environment first introduced in MultiCare's Cancer Center is now spreading to additional units. In her book, *Leading With Love*, Kathleen Sanford (1998) speaks about "leading oneself."[1] By this she means taking responsibility and caring for our own lives, not waiting for others, including management, to solve everything for us. All employees have a leadership responsibility in some form to help make the entire organization become successful.

We interviewed the following nurse executives and leaders:

▮ Kathleen Sanford, RN, DBA, Administrator (kathleensanford@hmh.westsound.net) and Vicki Enslow, RN, MN, Director Education Services, Harrison Memorial Hospital, Silverdale, Washington
▮ Pamela Bilbrey, MS, MBA, Senior Vice President of Corporate Development (pbilbrey@bhcpns.org), Baptist Health Care, Pensacola, Florida
▮ Kay Lanier, RN, BSN, MA, Clinical and Operations Director (kay.lanier @multicare.org), MultiCare Regional Cancer Center, Tacoma, Washington

- Colleen Person, BSN, RN, MMA, Vice President (cperson@chcm.com), Creative Health Care Management, Minneapolis, Minnesota
- Sharon Dingman, RN, BSN, MS, Consultant Specialist (sharondingman@aol.com), Creative Health Care Management, Ogden, Utah
- Inge Christensen, RN, MPH student, Teacher of Nursing, H:S School of Nursing, Copenhagen, Denmark (inch@mail.tele.dk)
- Sharon Rominger, RN, BS, MS, Nurse Executive and Director of Quality Initiatives (srominger@luhcares.org), Longmont United Hospital, Longmont, Colorado
- Colleen Goode, RN, PHD, FAAN, Vice President Patient Services & Chief Nursing Officer (colleen.goode@uch.edu) and Kathleen R. Smith, RN, MS, Informatics Nurse Specialist (kathy.smith@uch.edu), University of Colorado Hospital, Denver, Colorado

Their stories and insights are shared in three categories: The Role of Leadership, Education and Staff Development, and Models For Caring.

## The Role of Leadership

### A New Facility, A New Culture: Harrison Memorial Hospital

When Harrison Memorial Hospital in Bremerton, Washington, decided to build a second hospital some nine miles away in Silverdale, Kathleen Sanford, Vice President of Nursing Services, was tapped as its administrator. She realized that building a new facility gave management a tremendous opportunity to reshape the organization's culture and commitment to teamwork from the beginning.

"Hospitals often experience the problem of the silo effect, people not always working together as a team across functional lines," she states. "Everyone knows we are here to take care of patients, but we get into our professional groups and, because resources are limited, we tend to protect our turf. So we talk about teamwork, but in reality we don't often do it very well."

It becomes much more difficult to change an established culture as opposed to creating a fresh environment in a new organization, she explains. She wanted a culture where everyone knows from the beginning that his or her job is patient care and that everyone will work together as a team. Because many people do not really know what it means to be a "team," she defined it in specific terms of mutual support, communication, and accountability that were clearly stated even as the staffing process began.

"We were closing down some of our services in Bremerton and moving them to the new location, which in some areas meant job relocation. Everyone who potentially might move had to interview for his or her job, and the questions were very simple," she explains. "Technical competence was assumed, so the questions were structured to evaluate team competency. During meetings at the Bremerton hospital, prospective employee transferees were informed about the new Silverdale culture. Then, using specially designed questions, they were asked during the interviewing process whether they agreed with the teamwork concept as being concerned not only with the patient but also with their fellow workers."

After staffing was complete and before the doors were opened, Kathleen and her staff began an educational program to enhance people's skills in community building, nontechnical caregiving, communicating, problem solving, resolving conflicts, and maintaining high performance standards. "But," she asserts, "this wasn't just train them, leave them alone, then zap them when they fail to use these skills. Twice each year after the initial program, everyone in the hospital attends a daylong training event in addition to his or her clinical education. We continue to reinforce and grow the culture. We have even added a few new components, one of which involves healing related to personal psychological and emotional issues. Many healthcare providers are wounded healers in need of mending. So we help our employees to design personal self-care plans."

We asked Kathleen what she did to gain the support for a culture of caring from physicians. "When we want people to change, there must be something in it for them," she responds. "The growing nursing shortage became our opportunity to gain their attention. If we can't recruit and retain nurses, it is going to impact doctors' schedules and wallets. If there are no nurses, you cannot plan surgery and admit patients." Elaborating further, she explains, "There exists a small body of research on how physician behavior impacts employee morale, productivity, and retention. Of course, it's not the biggest reason for turnover, but it is a significant motivator, especially for people who have low self-esteem to begin with, who want to be cared for and admired. Doctors with lofty self-images and egos find it especially easy to abuse other staff personnel." One study by the VHA Inc., reported in the *American Journal of Nursing*, demonstrated that the quality of nurses' daily interactions with physicians had a major impact on their job satisfaction.[2] According to the study, 30% of nurses knew at least one nurse who resigned because of physician behavior.

Kathleen took the research finding to the hospital's medical executive committee, stating what support she needed from them, and received a remarkable, positive response. She claims it all has to do with the timing of the information, because the doctors could see the correlation between their practice interests and the impact of being a better team player on the welfare of the nursing staff.

## Core Leadership Competencies: Baptist Health Care

"Our leaders are trained to communicate to employees," states Pamela A. Bilbrey, Senior Vice President of Corporate Development at Baptist Health Care. "They are told, 'You are the CRO (Chief Retention Officer).' We want to make certain that each of our leaders understands the powerful relationship between the manager and the employee. It impacts productivity and longevity."

Pam reports that the organization has developed a list of 10 core competencies, each with behavioral descriptors, to identify and develop leaders. For example, the first item is "goal achiever," meaning that a person will set and share goals, establish high expectations, and motivate performance while instituting measurements. Leaders are held accountable through a 360-degree feedback instrument based upon the core competencies. Additionally, their leadership development program trains on these standards.

We questioned Pam about how this impacts diversity, because sometimes such standards create an environment in which most managers have similar personality traits. She responds, "All of our leaders complete the Myers-Briggs Type Indicator®, becoming well versed on the value of having a diverse workforce and how to pull teams together based upon individual strengths. Our training in this respect includes how to best communicate with different personalities. We also have a modified Myers-Briggs Type instrument that we use for all employees. Therefore, every leader gains a sense of the strengths of his or her employees and encourages the celebration of them."

Baptist holds its people accountable for achieving high standards of performance related to service excellence. This is just one example of why *Fortune* magazine selected the organization as fifteenth among the 100 best companies to work for in 2003.

The standards were developed by an employee team that looked at service excellence behaviors both within and outside of health care. They identified 10 standards that were verified by satisfaction surveys. All employees are expected to implement the following standards (one specific example of each standard is given):

▌ Attitude—Treat everyone as if he or she is the most important person in our facility.
▌ Appearance—Our dress always will be professional, tasteful, tidy, and discreet.
▌ Communication—Calls must be answered within three rings.
▌ Call Lights—All Baptist Hospital employees are responsible for answering patients' call lights.
▌ Commitment to Coworkers—Be supportive of fellow employees, offering help when possible.
▌ Customer Waiting—Offer refreshments and reading materials to waiting families.
▌ Elevator Etiquette—Smile and speak to fellow passengers.
▌ Privacy—Patients' records must be kept confidential.
▌ Safety Awareness—Report all accidents and incidents promptly and completely.
▌ Sense of Ownership—Use protective clothing and equipment when appropriate.

"Monthly, we celebrate and train to these standards," Pam asserts. "In addition, anyone applying for a job with Baptist Health Care must read our standards of performance booklet and sign an agreement to abide by them if hired. We believe this procedure sends a powerful message about how important these standards are to our culture."

She states that each month the organization celebrates one of the standards. "For example," she recounts, "if the standard has to do with commitment to coworkers, you can expect to find banners hung around the hospital, contests, word games, and other fun activities.

"People are held accountable by peers as well as their leaders. So, as part of our customer service, if someone looks lost in a hospital hallway, we don't just give him or her verbal directions, but actually walk them to their destination. If we fail to do so and an employee standing nearby observes it, she or he might say, 'Excuse me, but please remember our standards. If you are in a hurry going someplace else, perhaps I can help.'"

Baptist utilizes an *Engaged Selection* employment interviewing process. "Peer interviewing is very important in our organization," Pam underscores. "No person may be hired without having had at least two peer interviews, meaning that even the CEO cannot hire someone without feedback from others. This engagement practice increases our confidence in hiring the right person. For example, if I interview and select three candidates for a position reporting to me, at that time I turn them over to peer groups for interviewing. I visit with them to make sure they understand what the job entails, but I am not in the room when they actually conduct the interview. Afterward, they recommend one person who meets the criteria and the needs of the team."

Baptist also uses a suggestion program called *Bright Ideas.* It engages and empowers employees to make changes throughout the organization. The corporate goal of implementing 2.2 ideas per full-time employee in 2003 bears witness to how seriously they approach the program. Monthly, each leader provides a report regarding the organization's progress, and these reports are accessible to all leaders. In 2002, more than 8,000 bright ideas were implemented, and the estimated cost saving achieved exceeded more than $4 million.

Cascade Learning serves as an educational conduit throughout the Baptist Health Care organization. It flows from quarterly leadership development sessions involving some 500 leaders who supervise direct reports. Pam states, "One of our guiding principles entails the belief that leaders are teachers. If you attend one of these daylong quarterly sessions, you have a responsibility to share this information with your people. The knowledge level of the entire enterprise rises accordingly. To facilitate this and make it easier to pass the information along, we developed Cascade Learning Kits, a teaching tool containing scripts, quizzes, frequently asked questions, exercises, and the like. The leaders are held accountable for cascading the information to the troops within a period of 30 to 45 days."

Storytelling plays an important role at Baptist Health Care as one way of acknowledging employees. Stories flow through e-mails and surface during staff meetings. The organization circulates letters of appreciation from patients and posts accolades on communication boards. In addition, positive, nonmonetary feedback occurs through handwritten thank you notes usually mailed to employees' homes. Employees are aware that it is part of a manager's job responsibilities to write them every Friday afternoon, but they generate a lot of appreciation. "One young man phoned to thank an administrator for the letter sent to his mother, one of our employees," Pam informs us with enthusiasm. "He said that the family had the letter framed and hung it in their mother's living room."

Baptist Health Care annually publishes a booklet called *Legends*, sharing stories of outstanding service. For example, "Physical therapist, Nancy, visited the home of a man who did not want her services. During their discussion, he told her that he had no food, nor did he have any to give his dog. Nancy could have gone on to the next case, but instead went grocery shopping for him. When she returned, the man decided he did need home health services after all."

## Education and Staff Development

### Compassionate Communication: Harrison Memorial Hospital

Following the original mandatory orientation, Harrison Memorial Hospital, noted earlier in this chapter, made a commitment to conducting annual daylong follow-up workshops, part of a wellness initiative devoted to the caring side of the work going on there. According to Vicki Enslow, Director of Educational Services, each session begins with a general discussion of what is and what is not working. "We ask the question, 'Is this the best place you have ever worked? If so, why? And if not, why not?' We want people to identify any barriers to their calling and learn what the organization can do to respond."

The first follow-up event centered upon Compassionate Communication, a worldwide focus advancing nonviolent communication. Often, the language we are taught interferes with our desire to live in harmony with others and to care. Compassionate Communication eliminates the "shoulds" and "oughts" from language and emphasizes first-person terminology, such as "I think" or "I feel."

In 2002, the concept of a healing environment was introduced, an approach adapted from a model implemented in another healthcare facility. (More information on a Healing Environment can be found elsewhere in this chapter.) Employees were introduced to an optional self-care evaluation, which includes physical, emotional, and spiritual concerns and incorporates identifying personal growth goals, such as being trained in a specific modality like music or aromatherapy.

The underlining assumption in this focus on self-care is the belief that you cannot give something if you don't have it within yourself to give. "As a psychosocial nurse," Vicki asserts, "I have a strong belief that people need to develop a flexible boundary system. What is it that we really need to do for people, and what must they do for themselves? We need to give people the tools necessary for them to take care of themselves," she explains. "For example, we use the Kiersey Temperament Sorter II extensively throughout the hospital as a tool to increase meaningful communication and teamwork. The challenge is to maximize one's strengths and the strengths of those we work with to enhance the care of our customers."

## Cost Savings Through Staff Care: MultiCare Regional Cancer Center

Clinical and Operations Director Kay Lanier's journey toward creating a healthy, caring work environment began by exploring the question, "Can you teach caring?" During the process, she gained significant insight and support by joining the International Association for Human Caring. Through dialogue and collaboration with other nurses, she eventually came to believe that caring could be evoked by providing a safe and caring environment for the caregivers.

At the time Kay was asked to direct the Oncology Medical Surgical Unit in 1989, the cancer unit was troubled and felt unsupported by the organization. Because she was attempting to create an atmosphere almost unheard of in a healthcare inpatient environment, Kay launched a cultural transformation process by seeking out the best resources in psycho/social and spiritual care. She and her leadership team introduced change slowly and progressively to gain the staff's acceptance and support.

They began with a philosophy that recognizes the patient as the center of their awareness and holistic care. She affirms, "We believe that each person's life has meaning and that healing comes from within the individual. We treat the whole person and give control to him or her whenever possible. So often when people enter the hospital they lose control, so we wanted to change that. We also wanted to maintain the integrity of the human spirit and to decrease the suffering of body, mind, and spirit."

Surprisingly, and unlike many organizational enhancing initiatives, this was not a top-down initiative led by the organization's CEO. The overall hospital staff did not value the unit, and both nurses and patients expressed significant displeasure. "After a few years of listening and observing, it came down to the reality that the staff felt that no one cared for the nurses and valued them," she reports. "I sensed that if I cared for them, they would in turn care more holistically for the patients. Within a few years, our patient satisfaction ratings soared into the 90s, and our staff satisfaction skyrocketed as well, just by taking care of the nurses."

In addition to creating a pleasant, warm, and caring physical environment and adding clinical nurse specialists to ensure clinical competency among the newer employees, today leadership works to instill employees with integrity (meaning that words and actions match). They assist employees to balance body, mind, and spirit by:

▮ Employing a full-time, professionally trained counselor who spends at least 50% of her time with the staff;

▮ Providing training that includes communication skills, conflict resolution, teamwork, and leadership abilities;

▮ Offering a workshop through which employees explore their nonclinical work values and skills, leading to a heightened sense of purpose, self-care, and self-esteem.

As one might expect, this approach dramatically impacts the bottom line. In addition to almost always operating within budgetary perimeters, today the unit enjoys an RN vacancy rate of about 4.5% in contrast to the overall rate of 20% for the county. The American Organization of Nurse Executives' analysis indicates that it costs nearly $50,000 per registered nurse in visible and invisible turnover costs.

Kay asserts, "Research suggests that nurses come to the profession with an inherent sense of caring. Unfortunately, often they also come with limited conflict resolution skills and with low self-esteem, many having been raised in homes where they have not been valued. Once some of these factors have been eliminated or reduced, like a butterfly emerging from a cocoon, the caring begins to truly surface.

"For example, we had a nurse who acted like a brick wall surrounded her. You couldn't speak with her except clinically. She had experienced a very difficult family environment and had learned to protect herself from others. We did a lot of work with her, sending her to classes and encouraging her to work with our counselor. Today, she serves as one of the most caring people on our staff."

Again, Kay underscores, "We believe that if the employees are cared for, then patients will be cared for. A lot of organizations simply concentrate upon customer service and upon being nice to patients. Of course, there is nothing wrong with that, but it doesn't reach to the heart of the problem. We decided that we would begin by addressing the needs of the employee's heart as opposed to imposing some top-down dictated system."

Of course, many healthcare leaders might point to the expense of creating this kind of environment as being prohibitive. However, Kay informs us that for the first five years, they implemented their philosophy with no increase of money whatsoever. They simply utilized their own internal expertise. Then, in 1994, they received an endowment for nursing education from a local community foundation. They received $1 million to renovate the physical environment and provide staff educational opportunities, which was matched by the MultiCare organization.

When Kay and her staff interview for new nursing positions, they spend considerable time explaining the unit's philosophy. Once on the payroll, managers do not dictate behavior, but rather provide education as needed. Below is a sample of the leadership skills that Kay and her managers commit to utilizing. In addition, each year

---

### Sample of Caring Leadership Skills

▌ Listen in a nonjudgmental way.
▌ Tell the truth.
▌ Work as a team.
▌ Hold people accountable.
▌ Be flexible around change.
▌ Provide safety for staff in conflict situations.
▌ Have courage to confront in a caring way.
▌ Provide times of celebration.
▌ Walk the talk.
▌ Welcome feedback.

employees are asked to submit a self-care plan that is designed to help them maintain lifestyle balance and to aid in continued growth. The plan can be anything that they want it to be, but currently they are given a list of questions in seven categories. The following is a sampling of these questions:

| | |
|---|---|
| *Healing Environment* | How can you improve your contribution to the healing environment? |
| *Integrative Therapy* | What complementary/integrative therapies—meditation, massage, aromatherapy, music, therapeutic touch, etc.—do you use? What effect do they have? |
| *Meaning and Purpose* | What meaning and value does your work on our unit have in your life? |
| *Physical Balance* | What areas need improvement? |
| *Mental Balance* | How does your positive or negative energy influence the healing environment? |
| *Emotional Balance* | What emotions impede your being fully present to yourself and to others? |
| *Spiritual Balance* | What practices help you stay connected to your understanding of God? |

The idea is to visit with each employee and to determine how he or she wishes to grow in the coming year. What, if anything, seems to be out of balance? Kay shares an example, "Perhaps an employee wants to learn more about spiritual caregiving. Knowing this, we search out various resources and workshops, then recommend an activity using funds from our endowment."

We asked Kay whether the overall culture of the hospital made it more difficult to institute change and implement caring behaviors. She reports, "For a short while in the beginning, it did make it somewhat more difficult. However, we are now experiencing just the opposite effect. In addition to my current assignment, I have been asked by the CEO to assume leadership for another unit and to introduce a healing environment to it. The director of our hospice program who reports to me has requested that we help them as well."

Kay believes that today, most people invariably come to their work environments, health care or otherwise, with psychosocial wounds. Concerned, she declares, "Unfortunately, most organizations don't care to acknowledge these wounds or do anything to help people heal. Yet, it affects performance. We have a nurse whose child is suicidal and who may phone in sick several nights in a row. What should we do, punish her? Of course not! We do everything possible to support that person and to get her in touch with community resources. This, in turn, builds appreciation and loyalty. Caring begets caring, so we have a win-win situation for everyone."

### Reigniting Nursing Passion: Colleen Person

With nearly 40 years of nursing experience, Colleen Person, Vice President of Creative Health Care Management (CHCM), remains excited and passionate about her chosen profession. Today, as a consultant, she focuses her energies on strengthening relationships between nursing leaders and staff, between colleagues, and with staff and patients. "My work involves customizing consultation and education for organizations to develop leaders, staff, healthy interpersonal relationships, and effective communication," she states. "I facilitate organizations in identifying the principles associated with their vision and mission and turning them into intentional behaviors."

In a workshop entitled Re-igniting the Spirit of Caring, Colleen and her colleagues at CHCM call upon a variety of resources and exercises. Essentially, they focus on three dimensions: first, caring for self in terms of body, mind, and spirit; second, caring for colleagues; and third, caring for patients and their families. She also assists people in developing their own personal vision of their intention for their life and practice.

Colleen is an avid supporter of applying Appreciative Inquiry (AI) methodology. Each group event begins by asking participants to describe what they appreciate about their organization and/or the nursing profession in general. "It's amazing what happens when you shift the focus from being problem-oriented to sharing affirmations," Colleen avows. "The energy level skyrockets for both individuals and groups. As quantum science teaches us, energy flows in the direction to which we pay attention. We are known by the questions we ask. AI lays a collective foundation that is very important for positive organizational change.

"Then we move into the dimension of caring for self. We've always known about the long tradition in nursing of entering the profession in order to care for others. However, the sociological research shows us that many people in the helping professions engage in unhealthy relationships. Nurses in particular want to make a difference, yet some can be very needy themselves. In addition to reconnecting with what brings them to the profession, it is important to look at what happens in the work environment and to affirm and enhance healthy work environments.

"One of Kristen Swanson's five processes of caring is 'doing for.' It involves doing for people what they would do for themselves if they could. More important, nurses need to learn *not* to do for people what they can do for themselves. It's a generalization, but we tend to burn ourselves out when this caring activity goes beyond appropriate boundaries. It goes back to nursing education and needs identification. The more needs we identify and place in a care plan, the higher the grade we received. The task today must focus upon essential activities, creating a paradigm shift. We must ask:

- What do we need to continue to do for the patient?
- What do we need to do differently?
- What do we need to stop doing?"

According to Colleen, many nurses have sacrificed their souls for the sake of task-based caregiving, spending the majority of their time in mind-oriented thinking activities to the sacrifice of their physical health and spiritual well-being. "Given the demands of work, the number of nurses who ignore caring for their own bodies is staggering," she suggests. "The same holds true for spiritual and soulful values. In our workshops, we ask people to do one thing for themselves during the evening hours. The stories we hear the next morning would make you cry. People tell us that they have not taken time for themselves in years."

Colleen states that when people reconnect to why they entered nursing in the first place, there is a revitalization of their vision and values leading to taking care of others in a meaningful way. Rather than considering leaving the profession because of feeling burned out and tired, they say, "Now I remember why I became a nurse. It's all about relationships and about what I have to uniquely offer to people."

Colleen considers caring for colleagues equally important. She grins, "For years, the three 'Bs,' as we at CHCM call them, have been too prevalent in our profession—bickering, backbiting, and blaming. Nurses have so much to learn about how to function as colleagues," she says candidly. "It means developing mutual respect, trust, and open communication." She believes that utilizing an AI approach by sharing stories about times when people worked well together and what it would take to replicate that environment leads to a different perspective. By capturing themes, values, and behaviors, positive changes can occur in taking care of self and colleagues. One technique Colleen uses is to have people create a charter or use CHCM's "Commitment to My Coworker Card" that, instead of the three "Bs," identifies positive colleague behaviors, such as the three "Cs" of choosing, caring, and collaborating.

The third aspect of the caring foundation entails caring for patients and their families. Because personal experience is so important, Colleen notes, it is helpful to have people share their own experience, or that of a family member, of being cared for. "It makes the meaning of caring much more personal and less professionally detached," she believes.

Another helpful tool is creating a bridge to patient stories through a panel of patients sharing their experiences and the behaviors of caregivers that were most appreciated and what things they wish would have been done differently. "It becomes a rather rare feedback loop for the nurses; they don't often get to hear about the impact of their nursing activities," Colleen explains. "Often patients come to nurses at the most challenged times of their lives and nurses take that for granted. It tends to make concrete the importance of having eye contact, sitting in the presence of a patient, touching and asking what the patient needs."

Such an experiential process leads to a heightened awareness of the necessity of being interpersonally competent as well as technically competent. "By becoming reconnected with their values and calling, nurses are better able to translate the vision and values of the organization into behaviors with one another and with patients at a practical level. When they develop a personal vision for their life and practice and by re-connecting to the past, they can recommit to the future," she says firmly. "It is the wise organization that is investing in its staff, their most valuable resource. It costs an organization between $50,000 and $80,000 for each person who leaves. Just think how much organizations would save by retaining even one nurse! And just think what that means to that one nurse . . . to his or her patients and colleagues!"

### Nominal Group Technique: Inge Christensen

Inge Christensen serves in a full-time position teaching nursing and caring theory in Copenhagen, Denmark. She believes it is vital to begin focusing upon holistic patient care as early as possible in a nursing career, although the following methodology can be used with any group of seasoned nurses as well.

Inge defines caring as a way of being. "That is the ontological side of it. It is also a practice; caring is also something a person can learn to do and a science that can be explored. However, deep within us, caring is a way of being, and you would not become a nurse if you did not have such a desire to help others. It really is a calling."

When Inge served as a student advisor, she employed a methodology called "nominal group technique" as a way of introducing students at the start of their education to the concept of caring in the nursing profession using their own experiences in caring as human beings in general. This technique is a structured variation of small group discussion methods. The process prevents a single person from dominating the discussion, encouraging the more passive or silent group members to participate, and results in a set of prioritized solutions or recommendations. In the case of caring, the students developed their own very early model of the meaning of caring.

Students were placed in small groups, given sticky notes, and asked to write down thoughts and phrases they associate with caring. Inge asks two questions: "Think of a situation in which you felt cared for" and "think of a situation in which you did not feel cared for." Initially, they work individually without comment, writing their thoughts on sticky notes, and then they place their notes on a flip chart. They subsequently share their perceptions with the group about the nature of caring. Questions asking for clarification are allowed, but no criticism is permitted. The group then begins to structure the responses, eliminating duplications and combining them according to similarities. Finally, the list of characteristics is prioritized.

Inge affirms, "When you review the final product, it is awesome, because many of the core components on caring have been uncovered at a very early stage of the nursing education by the students themselves. The students stated that caring involves compassion, love, honesty, heart, openness, respect, trust, understanding, courage, presence, empathy, time, and use of intuition. The nurse has to be professionally skillful, competent, calm, a good listener, patient, able to quickly create an overview of the patients' situation and needs, engaged and interested in other human beings, and have a profound wish to help other human beings. Caring also involves supportive relatives, family, and friends of the patient and nurse, caring colleagues, and effective interdisciplinary collaboration.

"It compares quite favorably to Jean Watson's model of the 10 primary carative factors: those being the formation of humanistic–altruistic system of values; the instillation of faith and hope; the cultivation of sensitivity to one self and to others; the development of a helping and trusting relationship; the promotion and acceptance of the expression of positive and negative feelings; the systematic use of the scientific problem-solving method for decision making; the promotion of interpersonal teaching and learning; the provision for a supportive, protective, and/or corrective mental, physical, sociocultural, and spiritual environment; assistance with the gratification of human needs; and the allowance of existential–phenomenological forces. And it includes the transpersonal element. It embraces our connectedness and need for mutual caring. Also, I've found in working with different groups that almost every time they arrive at similar conclusions. It appears as though people instinctively know what it means to care. We all know how to care even though it may not be the focus of our attention. And often, the one's who do care center that interest in choosing to be nurses."

After completing the process, Inge encourages the students to use their creativity in making posters that display the meaning of caring. These are presented to fellow students of nursing and to students of other healthcare disciplines at cross-sectional conferences. At the very least, this process assists students in personalizing the theory of caring and in integrating it into their basic work orientation. Inge believes that it can become the first step toward a more conscious awareness of being uniquely called to care as a nurse, which in turn contributes to healing the whole person.

Beyond the school environment, this process could be used prior to introducing nursing research on the nature and processes of caring. A group could be asked to search for and to discuss similarities.

An alternate procedure might be to have people work in small groups to create a picture collage that depicts the nature of caring to be displayed somewhere in the unit as a visual reinforcement. Or this process could be used to have a nurse create a collage showing what self-care personally means to her or him.

## Models for Caring

### A Magnet Facility: University of Colorado Hospital

The University of Colorado Hospital in Denver received its Magnet designation from the American Nurses Credentialing Center in 2002. Colleen Goode, Vice President of Patient Services & Chief Nursing Officer (CNO), maintains, "Achieving it cannot simply be the goal of the CNO. You must solicit the support of the entire staff and explain why the designation is important. Kathy Smith [Informatics Nurse Specialist] and I worked on this together for about 18 months, gaining the commitment of a large group of people before we actually applied." They believe that the designation was important not only for the staff but for patient outcomes as well.

"We have periodic retreats for our executive team," states Colleen. "At one of them, we brainstormed some rather far-reaching five-year goals. One of mine related to achieving Magnet status. As an executive group, we actually voted on the goals because it was important to get a commitment in terms of energy and resources. There was unanimous support for working toward the Magnet designation."

The Magnet label designation came about in the 1980s during the nursing shortage. Studies determined that some hospitals in the same geographic area as others did not experience any shortage. What was it about these hospitals that favorably influenced nurse retention? Essentially, the research demonstrated that when nurses feel good about themselves, feel rewarded, remain proud of their work environment, and believe they can give good patient care, they tend to remain with the organization. When facilities seek Magnet status, personnel are invited to conduct an evidence-based evaluation of whether the hospital meets certain criteria of excellence. Broadly speaking, it entails creating an atmosphere of work satisfaction and nurse empowerment.

"In looking at the criteria, we realized that we had all of the various components already in place," Colleen explains. "It became a matter of strengthening them. For example, one of the areas we worked on building up had to do with cultural diversity. Educational opportunities were somewhat limited in terms of providing culturally sensitive care. Although already part of our orientation program, it needed to be updated. We also installed a mandatory course attended by the entire staff."

A significant number of the nurses at the hospital have received some of their education through Dr. Jean Watson, currently Distinguished Professor at the Health Science Center School of Nursing, and consequently have been exposed to her caring theory. Kathy Smith states, "Applications of her theory permeate much of our patient care. Not only do they obtain their bachelor's degree at the Health Science Center, but many of them also go there for advanced degrees as well. Colleen very much supports Jean's work. She serves as an advocate for the nurses, respecting their worth, listening to them, and encouraging their development."

Much of the hospital's environment is relationship based. Colleen asserts, "In our leadership team, you will find a group of people who truly care about each other and who support each other's respective tasks. This includes having fun and getting involved socially. In addition, we give our nurses at the unit level a great deal of autonomy in making decisions about how the unit operates, administratively as well as clinically."

Colleen believes that leaders who are visible and available impact the organization more than anything else. She schedules rounds on her calendar, giving staff nurses an opportunity to communicate on the unit level. "I have to demonstrate that I care about them. They want me to know about their issues. Actually, our entire leadership team saturates the organization with their presence, including the CEO.

"Another concrete way we care for our people is through honoring experience," Colleen underscores. "We have a clinical ladder of progression that recognizes excellence and gives people an opportunity to advance while remaining at the bedside. It empowers nurses as well as impacting their salary. Many other hospitals contact us for information and advice about it.

"We also have a strong preceptor program that serves to monitor and promote clinical excellence. We have a training program for preceptors on how to teach staff and give constructive feedback. Because turnover rates tend to be very high among new graduates, even more important is our strong orientation program for new graduating nurses. Because of the very ill patients they see here, it would be very hard for them to enter our environment without it."

Kathy affirms this, adding, "This is one of the main reasons for our one-year residency program for nurses. In addition to enhancing their clinical skills, they learn how to communicate with patients and physicians. Part of the program involves a pilot demonstration project entitled *Caring for Yourself*. We provide information about balancing work and family life. We train nurses how to care for themselves and support colleagues at the unit level."

A number of the nursing units have identified specific behaviors surrounding self-care and patient care, including some of the physicians. "For example, one of the surgical intensive units focuses upon collaborative practice," Kathy informs us. "Evidence-based research indicates that patient outcomes in intensive care units improve when nurses and physicians work as a collaborative team. We have courses on communication, collaboration, and the like taught through our human resources department. Courses for managers are mandatory."

From four years ago to present, the hospital's turnover rate dropped from about 18% annually to 7%. Colleen and Kathy believe that having the Magnet designation contributes to this trend because nurses desire to work in this kind of environment. The hospital uses very few agency or traveling nurses, unusual for the Denver area.

Both Colleen and Kathy believe that most people enter the nursing profession because of an interest in a service-oriented profession, desiring to really make a difference in people's lives though their daily work. Today, nursing attracts people who are very intelligent, especially because the patients cared for in hospitals are more acutely ill. Along with teachers, nurses have a huge impact upon people's lives.

Acknowledging some of the negative external forces that exist in health care today, the regulatory issues, limited resources, and the long hours, Colleen replies, "Again, the most important factor in our environment is the belief that nurses are important and should feel valued. They know that their role remains vital in someone's recovery from illness, and everyone respects them for it. You will find little or no 'It's us against them' attitudes among nurses, administrators, or doctors.

"We are also very protective in our nurse/patient ratios. Nothing drives nurses away faster than if they cannot provide the care that they feel the patient needs. Our ratios on our medical/surgical unit are 4 to 1 on the day shift and 5 to 1 at night."

One of the arguments for increasing patient load per nurse stems from economic considerations as well as from nurse shortages. "Actually," Kathy states, "If you have high ratios that lead to high turnover, resulting in an increased use of agency and traveling nurses, it becomes extremely expensive. It costs more than if you have low ratios. We are doing every bit as well financially as those people with high ratios."

Caring is part of the hospital's culture. Colleen explains using an example. "When answering the telephone or when speaking to any group in the hospital, we introduce ourselves, 'I am Mary Jones and I am a member of the [department] care team.' So, caring is embedded in our language."

Agreeing, Kathy states, "Every day we ask ourselves what barriers stand in the way of genuinely caring for ourselves, our colleagues, patients, and their families. Then we do everything possible to remove them. For example, in our emergency department, we established an initiative that when a person needs to be admitted, that patient will be in a hospital bed within one hour. That becomes a very challenging task, but it serves as an example of our commitment and courage to care."

## A Planetree Affiliate Facility: Longmont United Hospital

Sharon Rominger, Nurse Executive and Director of Quality Initiatives at Longmont United Hospital, Colorado, knows firsthand the opportunities provided by the nursing profession in moving from the bedside to the administrative side of health care. She began a career that spans almost 40 years as a medical/surgical nurse technician, went on to obtain her associate degree followed by her RN degree, and later earned her master's degree as a Clinical Nurse Specialist. She remains as passionate about her work now as in the beginning. She is especially enthusiastic about working in a facility that is a Planetree affiliate, which prides itself on providing an innovative mix of music, art, architecture, and technology ministering to the body, mind, and spirit. Eyes twinkling, she proclaims, "I have a fairy tale story of how this hospital takes care of its people and how it became a Planetree affiliate."

In 1997, Sharon and several other staff members heard about Planetree during a Colorado Hospital Association conference. "We said to each other, 'In general, that describes us, but we could really build upon our strengths if we implemented it.' Located in a small community, we always cared for people well, because in many instances, we knew them as neighbors. However, we believed the Planetree approach to 'humanize, demystify, and personalize care' would bring our caring to a new level. It also caused us to state concretely that we would care for the body, mind, and spirit. So we decided to enter a process of transformation, elevating patient and employee caring to a much higher level."

The first step in the process involved developing an orientation program for all employees, which was actually conducted by the CEO and division directors. It included positive attitude enhancement and service recovery. Today, all new employees attend a similar orientation. "Service recovery" means meeting the needs of patients while they are in the hospital, because this is the best time to recover their allegiance.

In order to not only meet a patient's immediate needs, but to go the extra mile, Sharon relates, "Looking through the eyes of the patients, we initiated a 20-20 'vision' program. We commit to giving our employees 20 minutes and/or $20 to please a patient. It allows staff to initiate creative and forward thinking activities as well as to take quick action if there are complaints. For example, someone's magazines may have been removed during cleaning, and when that patient returns from a procedure, he or she wonders what happened to them. So, the nurse is preauthorized to go to the gift shop, purchase new magazines, and put the expense on the 20-20 tab. Also, patient representatives visit every new patient daily.

"The hospital encourages innovation," she underscores. "Managers are trained to respond enthusiastically about an idea before expressing any concerns about it." Although Sharon did not use the words *itemized response*, the intent is the same, which is to respond to an idea with two or three things you like about it before mentioning any possible pitfalls related to its implementation.

Longmont also instituted "administrative rounding." Each week an administrator "rounds" in the facility to see if there are any issues needing to be addressed. In addition, if any kind of urgent event or crisis is in the wind, administrators return to the hospital during the evening or on weekends to help out. This approach alleviates the perceived gap between staff and administration.

Sharon underscores the importance of caring in health care, emphasizing, "I truly believe that caring represents the essence of nursing. If it's not, we are in trouble because nurses are at the bedside 24 hours a day, seven days a week. We interact with patients at their most vulnerable times, from birth to death. What I like the most about the Planetree model is its emphasis upon human interaction. With the rapid proliferation of medical technology, much of whole-person human relations have diminished. Institutions changed nursing through their emphasis upon the medical model and not the nursing model.

"The medical model tends to be production oriented, so I ask every group of new nurses to describe their heart's desire and hope for their careers when they graduated from school. Then I ask what is keeping or might keep them from doing it. I want to leave Longmont knowing that we have caring nurses unbridled by institutional technocratic indifference. For example, when we built a new addition to the hospital, we involved the nurses in the design and attempted to remove any barrier between the nurse, the patient, and the family. Physically and otherwise, we place nurses in the position of not simply caring, but of managing patient care. Our staff nurses orchestrate the care in collaboration with the other disciplines.

"Another example is what we describe as 'rounding,'" Sharon continues. "When the shift changes, both nurses visit the patient's room and report one to the other in front of the patient so that the patient becomes part of the loop. I've been working on this technique for a long time, and it makes a huge difference. The nurse also joins the physician when he or she is in the room speaking to the patient so that the nurse can later reinforce the doctor's communication."

In terms of some of the "softer" aspects of caring, the hospital brought in the original Patch Adams to spend time with the staff. He clowned around for both the staff and the patients. One of the volunteers who was a professional clown took over after he left. She and other individuals established a healthcare clown college, teaching others how to clown for both children and adults.

"Art the Cart" is another innovative idea that has been introduced. The cart is filled with artistic supplies and, based upon the patient's situation and need, the art therapist suggests different art approaches for both children and adults. Various art forms also dominate the physical environment.

On a pay-as-you-go basis, additional complementary therapies are available through the hospital, including music therapy, massage therapy, reflexology, acupuncture, and other Eastern-oriented modalities. The director of these services currently reaches a community audience of more than 2,000 people. Every new mother receives a massage. At times, services such as a massage are available for free to employees as a reward for outstanding work. Or a manager may buy a massage for a staff member who seems particularly stressed. Finally, as appropriate, the hospital allows animals to join the patients. One such occasion was chronicled in a book of stories Longmont publishes periodically.

> An 86-year-old woman was allowed to sleep next to her spouse of nearly 60 years during his last hours of life. He passed away in his wife's arms with his dog asleep near the foot of the bed.

"We offer a Planetree Retreat to specific departments and their employees," Sharon explains. "People identify all of the barriers existing in their unit and implement changes whenever possible. The Planetree philosophy states that the entire organization needs to be cared for, but specific units may have particular needs.

"The retreat concept along with other Planetree strategies contributes greatly to nurse retention. During the last three years," states Sharon, "the nursing turnover rate dropped from about 30%, average for this part of the country, to about 6% per year."

Not surprisingly, Sharon utilizes the physical environment and the overall concept of being a Planetree facility as a recruiting tool. She says, "I know that nurses truly want to care for patients, so I personally take prospective nurses on a tour of our facilities. I let the atmosphere as well as our employees bear witness to our mission, vision, and values. Hiring a nurse is very easy after such an orientation," she says with a smile.

Basically, Longmont identified its strengths and then asked itself, "How can we build upon them?" As mentioned elsewhere in this book, they serve as a prime example of the intervention technique called Appreciative Inquiry, identifying what an organization does well and then systematically embellishing it.

### The Caring Model™: Sharon Dingman's Synthesis of Caring Theories

Sharon Dingman's personal experience, first as a patient with an extended, complicated hospital stay, and second, years later as the Chief Nursing Officer/Chief Operating Officer in a rural, 49-bed hospital, ultimately led to the creation and development of The Caring Model™.[3] In 1979, Sharon experienced an initially undiagnosed perforated appendix, which eventually culminated in surgery. However, she developed gangrene, necessitating a second surgery. She recalls lingering near death for about three days. During her hospital stay, she experienced caring at its best and at its worst. Recognizing the importance of caring on a personal level led Sharon to return to school in 1980 to enter a nursing career. Caring and making a difference became her passions.

At the time of her CNO/COO experience, she recounts, management observed a decline in the "very satisfied" scores of patient satisfaction as measured by a Gallup Corporation survey. Problems especially surfaced in the areas of staff anticipating patient needs, responding to requests, communicating effectively, explaining procedures, and calming fears. According to Sharon, people often recommend hospitals by the care they receive. "Satisfaction with care is largely based on the perceptions of the caregiver's affective behavior toward the patient, family, and other caregivers," she states. Care includes nurses' attitudes, their promptness, cheerfulness, ability to calm fears, and ability to communicate clearly.

The identification of "critical junctures" in delivering care or service was explored. "We found that patients most often were more likely to forgive an unfortunate outcome than forgive a lack of concern and a lack of communication (excluding problems related to safety or mistakes) if they felt that the staff really cared about them. We also determined that patients could tell if the staff really enjoyed where they worked and whether their behaviors were congruent with the organization's stated and communicated mission and values. People can see what occurs at the nurse's station or in the halls and whether there exists a general sense of camaraderie," Sharon recounts. "We wanted to assess caring among colleagues as well as how caring behaviors impact patients' perceptions and satisfaction.

"There is a cascade effect," states Sharon. "Dissatisfied employees lead to unhappy patients and families and, in turn, to disgruntled physicians, and that may influence physicians' admissions and employers directing people to the hospital. So, if any unit of the caring team becomes disgruntled and detached, it impacts the whole organization, the patient, the family, and, ultimately, the bottom line and market share," she says emphatically.

Sharon's model integrates the caring theories of Kristen Swanson, Jean Watson, and Madeliene Leininger, as well as the key features of her own approach to caring activities. The specific emphasis incorporated from each includes:

- Swanson—Maintaining belief, knowing, being with, doing for, enabling/informing;
- Watson—Dignity, worth, and uniqueness of the individual, movement toward life purpose/completion, mutual human-to-human caring;
- Leininger—Care is essential for human growth and occurs when cultural values and practices are known and used explicitly;
- Dingman—Personal communication and accountability—introducing oneself and explaining one's role, using a patient's preferred name, maintaining eye and

touching contact, saying thank you coupled with the ability to articulate and live in congruence with the vision, mission, and values of the organization.

The basic tenets of Sharon's The Caring Model™ are:

▌ It is a practical approach to improving satisfaction, care, and outcomes;
▌ The set of five specific behaviors provides a framework for a renewed emphasis upon caring:

1. Introduce yourself to patient/family/client and explain your role in their care or service for that day.
2. Call the patient by his or her preferred name.
3. Use touch appropriately, a handshake or touch on the arm.
4. Direct patient caregivers to sit at the patient's bedside for at least 5 minutes per shift to plan and review the patient's care. Nondirect caregivers share information about procedures, processes, or services involved in attaining a desired outcome.
5. Use the mission, vision, and value statements of the organization in the patient's care plan.

▌ It identifies the "critical junctures" at the unit and organizational level to improve service and care;
▌ It promotes the strengthening of the infrastructure around initiatives;
▌ It offers visible leadership support of action;
▌ It encourages improved interpersonal relationships through building trust with open and honest communication; and
▌ It is quantifiable by using current organizational data to measure outcome indicators.

The model was introduced to hospital employees through two-and-a-half-hour training sessions with a primary goal of creating an emotional connection for the caregiver to the essence of caring. An organizational enhancement methodology called Appreciative Inquiry was used to help participants focus upon positive caring events in their lives as opposed to uncaring situations. People shared caring stories about what brought them into a healthcare profession and about what caring might mean from the point of view of the patient. Sharon maintains, "The majority of people who enter health care want to do a good job, and many of them feel called to their profession. We experienced an atmosphere of celebration by emphasizing what employees are doing well.

"I always share real stories about my feelings," she says, recounting two stories related to her hospital experience noted earlier. "I remember coming out of the second surgery, not being able to swallow well, but being able to hear two men talking over me. One of them was discussing an upcoming exam that would lead to a good position. One finally remarked that he needed to insert a catheter. 'I haven't done a female catheter in years!' he said. I don't remember much after that, but I do know they were discussing me, the female. This was in the days before I was a nurse, so I really didn't know what was going on."

Sharon's second story is a testimony to the circle of care. "During my hospital stay, I had a CNA, Maria, who was wonderfully considerate. She not only helped me, but also supported me by encouraging me in what I could do for myself. Nine years later as a nurse, I cared for her in the end stages of chronic obstructive disease, and I was with her when she died."

Any organizational and systematic issues that surfaced during the training sessions were placed on an "opportunity" list and given to a steering committee specifically formed to address such issues. When some session feedback suggested the perception that front-line employees exhibit caring behaviors but not managers, the model was expanded to include caring manager-training sessions. In part, leadership training focused on the importance of having clear role expectations and responsibilities. Managers are expected to show employees the same caring behaviors that are expected for patients and their families. Healthy caring and compassionate service evolve from caring and compassionate leaders.

Leadership responsibilities included:

▮ Creating and maintaining an enthusiastic caring environment;
▮ Assuring that caring expectations were known and acted upon. Philosophy and behaviors needed to be included in job descriptions, performance reviews, and documentation processes;
▮ Building an environment in which people feel accountable for their work and feel good about what they are doing;
▮ Helping to resolve critical issues; and
▮ Celebrating moments of excellence.

Sharon reports that outcomes were positive.[4] Three months after the intervention, two of the eight attributes from the Gallup Patient Satisfaction Survey originally studied were found to have a significantly higher rating. Unsolicited complaints remain low, including complaints from physicians. Employees saw managers exhibiting behaviors that support caregiving. They felt that their opinions counted and that their work made a difference. Collegiality remained high, and opportunities for celebration continue to take place.

Today, as a consultant with a national healthcare management firm, Sharon continues using the model. Much of her ongoing work revolves around helping others understand the significance of caring as an important indicator to measure the quality of care and to the financial success of the healthcare organization. "Caring behaviors must be broadly applied to all employees of the organization as well as to patients and their families," she states emphatically.

# Caring for Your Nursing Career

Career counseling professionals often use four words to describe work: job, career, mission, and calling. They can be visualized in the form of a triangular hierarchy as shown below. To a degree, they relate to Abraham Mazlow's famous hierarchy of needs that, starting from the bottom and working upward, are:

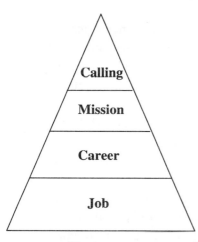

4. Esteem: Competence, meaning, purpose
3. Community/Belonging: Being accepted
2. Safety/Security: Out of danger
1. Physiological: Hunger, thirst

Having a *job* stands at the base of the triangle and pertains to physiological and safety needs. A job provides the basic needs of food and shelter, but often provides little in the way of self-fulfillment. A person may be forced to work for a minimum wage, also causing a sense of reward to be negligible. If a person won the lottery, he or she might walk away singing, "Take this job and shove it."

Having a *career* may bring with it a higher sense of safety and security, along with financial reward and success. A career may carry a heightened sense of acceptance and prestige in the eyes of the public, coupled with a sense of belonging to a fairly elite group of people. Nonetheless, at times when the external environment changes, one's sense of self-fulfillment may become diminished, as it did for some lawyers in the early 1990s and for some physicians in the late 1990s.

*Mission* implies a sense of dedication to a cause, such as Mothers Against Drunk Driving or Physicians For Social Responsibility. Committing to a higher cause often gives meaning and purpose to work. Unfortunately, often meaning and purpose bring little or no financial reward or much success in eliminating social problems, such as drinking while driving or nuclear proliferation.

Career guidance professionals usually reserve the word *calling* for the highest level of work. While often associated with a call to ordained ministry, it is not necessarily limited to religion. In his book *Callings: Finding and Following an Authentic Life*, Greg Levoy (1997) discusses methods to invoke calling into one's life, using art, pilgrimage, myth, and memory to help it to emerge into consciousness. He proclaims, "The purpose of calls is to summon adherents away from their daily grinds to a new level of awareness, into a sacred frame of mind, into communion with that which is bigger than themselves."[5]

In *The Soul's Code*, James Hillman (1996) confirms the belief that people carry a destiny within their psyches.[6] He states that, just as an acorn instinctively knows how to become an oak tree, so we have a calling. Where recognized or actualized, all humans have an exceptional component to their lives. When investigated and brought to consciousness, at least in part, it brings self-fulfillment, meaning, and purpose into being.

In *Hearing With The Heart*, Debra Farrington (2003) validates this by speaking of gifts. "Gifts are those abilities that seem to arise within you without any training or conscious development. Perhaps they are even inborn."[7]

For many years, Martha Finney and Deborah Dasch (1998) has been researching and writing about the work of ordinary people. In *Find Your Calling, Love Your Work*, Martha reports, "When you marry skills, passions, and experiences, you produce a life for yourself that is larger, easier, and more effective than you could have dreamed of in all your years struggling in mismatched jobs."[8]

Often, the biggest obstacle to consummating this marriage is an inner voice saying we are "supposed to." You are supposed to earn a living and not follow your heart's desire. You are supposed to remain in a mismatched job because it offers security. Work is drudgery and you are not supposed to enjoy it. You are supposed to retire at age 65 and not continue having a productive work life.

Although not a random sample, we interviewed more than 60 nurses and doctors for this book and *The Soul of the Physician* (2002). Many of them reported being attracted to their professions almost from the start. Feedback from his sixth-grade teacher planted a seed that germinated over time for Don Greggain, MD. "By the time I actually applied to medical school, I did believe that I was born to be in medicine."[9] Lon Hatfield, MD, speaks about awesome, mysterious "morphogenic fields" pulling us into conscious awareness. He reports, "When I was 12 years old, I wrote a paper on what I would be when I grew up, and it involved the general practice of medicine."[10]

Home care nurse Dee Horn's calling came to consciousness as a candy striper. "They gave me a gold charm that was a nurse's cap and said that I needed to enter nursing because it appeared to be my calling," she reveals. Parish nurse Joan Purdon informs us, "My dad was a Lutheran minister. I often went with him on Sunday afternoons to the hospital while he visited the sick. I remember enjoying just sitting in the lobby and soaking up the hospital atmosphere while he made his rounds."

Whether you care to use words like career, mission, or calling, meaningful, purposeful, and satisfying work emerges from entering a process called *discernment*. The word derives from the Latin *discernere*, meaning to "separate apart." All of us are multiskilled individuals, possessing a range of from 300 to 500 abilities, everything from driving a car to writing an e-mail. In fact, data on various occupations indicate that nurses are especially multitalented, not only clinically, but also in many other ways. They can be entrepreneurs, artists, educators, record keepers, counselors, managers, mechanics, and much more. The challenge is to separate the wheat from the chaff, identifying skills (or what Farrington calls gifts) that bring significant satisfaction and joy into one's life as well as contributing to the greater good.

In the chapter about Sandi Harding, she suggests a discernment image of "coming beside another person," knowing that we cannot enter the skin of that person to know completely her or his experiences, thoughts, and feelings. It entails taking the time to learn about a person without passing judgment, looking into someone's situation and discerning what is needed.

The Quakers have a special technique called a Clearness Committee. It is used as a way for a person seeking clarity of vision on an issue to gain from the wisdom of a group. Members of the committee have only one option: that of posing questions. They may not offer advice or opinions, make judgments, or even "follow up" on responses made to previous questions. The assumption is that, if they aren't bombarded with other peoples' advice, expertise, and even well-meaning suggestions, the individual will arrive at his or her own insight and/or solution.

Our distinctive, passionate gifts are often as close to us as the nose on our faces. But like our nose, we cannot see it very well without a mirror. Therefore, if you are interested in gaining more clarity regarding your career direction and calling, we now provide you with the following strategies and exercises.

## Parental Influence on Careers

With respect to work, what was your father's main advice (or that of another significant male in your life), either spoken verbally or nonverbally through his actions? Your mother's main advice? Because we were dependent upon them for survival, our parents and other significant adults had tremendous influence upon us when we were children. We carefully paid attention to what they said and did, and we carry their messages and scripts into adulthood often unconsciously. In terms of vocation, if these messages are congruent with and supportive of innate skills and abilities, then they help us to achieve satisfying ends in terms of career direction. If not, they may lead us down tragic, dysfunctional paths. Identifying them is the first step toward embarking on a more fulfilling path.

Listed below are some common assumptions about work, at least for those of us raised in earlier generations. Have you heard any of them coming from the lips of your parents or other significant adults in your life?

"Work for the golden age of retirement."
"After this reorganization, things will go back to normal."
"A good day's work will keep you on the payroll."
"Be practical and do something that will pay the bills."
"You can't afford to change jobs after 40."
"By their very nature, some jobs are secure."

For example, Jim's father said, "work hard, be responsible, and you'll get ahead." He was an electrical engineer who progressed to become a division superintendent in a utility company. Jim admired his father, so when it came time to choose a college major, he decided upon electrical engineering. Although graduating with this degree, it became apparent to him that he would be, at best, mediocre in this profession. He then entered the ministry and became a parish pastor for 10 years. Still motivated to "get ahead" like his father, he entered a career transition program and eventually secured a job in a utility company as a training specialist. Unconsciously following his father's unspoken vocational advice, he progressed to the point of becoming a training manager. Fortunately, at least in part, this career was aligned with his innate skill cluster of *optimizing* and his specific skill of *synthesizing*.

### Rearview Mirror Exercise

This strategy may require considerable time and reflection. Review your past life and identify four or five peak experiences from various ages. These were the special occasions in your life when a project or activity seemed almost effortless and engaged your energies. What special gifts or skills emerged during this time, bringing a deep sense of satisfaction and accomplishment? It is helpful to write a paragraph about these peak experiences, then look for patterns of skills. To help bring some of these events to consciousness, as mentioned in the chapter on strategies and resources, we highly recommend the resource book *A Guide for Recalling and Telling Your Story* (Hospice Foundation of America, 800-854-3402). Questions such as "What are your favorite memories about school?" help you to look into the rearview mirror of your life.

Along these lines, one of Shoshone nurse Naomi Mason's skill clusters involves *learning*. "I am an innately curious person," she reports. "We raised a lot of chickens and when one of them died prematurely, I would open it up and try to find the cause." As a child, Janet Hersh informs us, "Whenever someone in the family became ill, I would run and put it on [her Halloween nurse's uniform] and pretend to be a nurse." One of her key skill clusters is *compassion*.

On the other hand, occasionally a vocational calling will emerge from negative experiences. Sister Peggy Fannon recalls, "When I was four years old, I was taken to the hospital because of numerous ear infections. From that time on, all I ever talked about was being a nurse." Diane Newman found herself eventually called to cardiac nursing because "My Dad had a heart attack and we've had 10 uncles who died from them."

### Establish and Participate in a Speaking Event

Invite five or six friends to join you for one or more storytelling sessions. Each person takes the stage and offers a five-minute spontaneous talk about what he or she enjoys most about life in general and specifically in work (including unpaid work).

Afterward, each person gives positive feedback regarding perceptions of the person's skills and interests. If you get to do this over and over again during several sessions, a pattern will emerge, and your strengths will be anchored more concretely in your consciousness.

## Pay Attention to Your Words

In particular, career counselors discipline themselves to pay special attention to certain words such as *love* or *enjoy*. These serve as clues in identifying passionate interests and skills. For example, during our interview, Diane Newman revealed, "I love a challenge. Tell me that it can't be done and I will do my best to get it done. It's become my challenge to both my friends and patients, my motto, saying to them, 'You can do it!'" Nursing professor Carolyn Cagle said she "thoroughly enjoys helping people become quality parents."

Career counselors also listen for repetitious words and phrases. While interviewing parish nurse Sandi Harding, we noted the number of times she spoke about "coming beside" and "engaging" another person. In one form or another, during our conversion, home care nurse Marianne Davis used the word *analyze* several times, also identifying it is a key, passionate skill.

On the other hand, another exercise is to focus attention on the "flip side." What words do you use to express strong dislikes? On one side of a piece of paper, make a list of them in terms of distasteful activities, then on the right side turn each negative into a positive opposite. Sister Peggy Fannon strongly dislikes detailed work such as budgeting. She is a big-picture person who is more interested in possibilities.

Another way to understand "paying attention" entails engaging in "active receptivity." What it doesn't mean is, so to speak, sitting passively in a chair and waiting for enlightenment to come upon us in the form of a calling. Rather, we must be active in the sense of engaging in daily work (paid or otherwise) and in utilizing the strategies and tools listed in this chapter. Receptivity involves being attentive to the patterns that emerge over time, trusting the process as we actively seek direction, and remaining receptive to the events of the days and weeks ahead of us.

## Pay Attention to Your Body

Healthcare providers are trained to pay attention to the body. However, the body also informs us of stress reactions when we are engaged in dissatisfying work. Then too, it relays pleasant feelings of joy and peaceful integration when we engage our gifted skills.

Again, in *Hearing With The Heart*, Debra Farrington lists several exercises to listen to the body. Keep a journal of how your body feels in the morning, during meal times, and before bed. What events cause stress and what activities bring feelings of excitement? Notice the patterns as you continue logging your experiences during the week.

Especially when faced with two difficult and conflicting choices, make a list of all of the pros and cons related to each choice. Then, make a decision based upon a coin toss. For example, you may be conflicted between remaining in your current job and seeking new employment. If the coin lands "heads," you will remain; if it turns up "tails," you will leave. Now, observe your body. How does it feel? If you feel relaxed and relieved, then implement your decision announced by the coin. If you feel nervous and tense, delay the decision and work on expanding your options before taking a final step. The wisdom of the body is one of our greatest advocates.

### Talk to Your Guardian Angel

Picture the little girl holding the hand of an angel in *City of Angels*. She dies, and walking down the hallway hand in hand with the angel, she is asked, "What did you like best about your life?" How would you answer the question? Again, look through the rearview mirror of your life. So far, what have you liked best about your work life (paid or unpaid)? What one problem were you born to solve? Or what opportunity were you placed on earth to address?

### Take Yourself to the Bookstore

Take yourself on a trip to the bookstore, observing yourself entering and moving toward a particular section. What general categories draw your interest? What titles interest you? What magazines interest you? If you could write a book, it would be about what subject? What general arena of knowledge represents an opportunity of lifelong learning for you?

### Whose Job Do You Want?

Live the question as you continue through the days and weeks and observe people in the news or in your work environment. Recall Sandi Harding's story about sitting in a pool on a sunny day when the subject of parish nursing came up. She proclaimed, "That's it!" Consult the Want Ads. Conduct information interviews, determining what education and skills are required. By utilizing a search engine such as www.google.com, a wide array of information may be available on any given subject or occupation. A number of college career centers offer free Internet on-line information and exercises. In addition, you might visit Sigma Theta Tau International's web site (www.nursing-society.org) and peruse their excellent "Career Map" section.

## *Two Instruments, One Goal: Finding the Gifts of You*

Many of the nurses interviewed for this book completed the following two instruments. The Skill Clusters Inventory identifies 30 generic sets of skills. The Transferable Skills Card Sort offers more than 60 specific, nonclinical skills. Complete these instruments by following the directions, then look for patterns and complementary skills. Share the results with friends and colleagues. You might invite them to reflect upon the results, which can provide valuable, positive feedback.

As you begin to work with the instruments, keep in mind the following criteria for identifying and evaluating skills that serve as your most enjoyable gifts:

- Time flies when you are using this skill;
- This skill conjures up enthusiasm (a word that means "in God");
- This skill brings with it the use of joyful concentration;
- This skill is something you *cannot not* do;
- On a daily basis, this skill is used as the path of least resistance;
- Using this skill energizes you; and
- You learn easily when using this skill.

## Skill Clusters Inventory

A skill cluster contains a number of specific, observable skills that are closely related to one another. (For example, the *learning* cluster embraces a range of specific skills such as reading, questioning, and researching.) Identifying these clusters more clearly enhances our sense of purpose and direction in life. By following the instructions given at the end of this inventory, you will be able to identify a prioritized list of some of your key, satisfying clusters.

## Skill Clusters

**Analytical:** Using mental processes to explore reasons and causes. Looking before you leap

**Naturist:** Orienting toward physical nature, outdoor activities, and adventure

**Idea-oriented:** Freethinking and gravitating toward new ideas and possibilities

**Conviction:** Steadily maintaining a core set of beliefs and values

**Compassion:** Understanding and empathizing with others

**Communication:** Articulating thoughts and feelings. Listening effectively. Writing well

**Service/Dedication:** Teaching, helping others, making the world a better place

**Pure challenge:** Doing the impossible, desiring to compete and win

**Historic:** Researching the past and learning from it

**Entrepreneurship:** Starting a new venture, overcoming obstacles, and taking risks

**Acceptance:** Getting along with people and bringing them together

**Achievement-oriented:** Working hard with tenacity to achieve results

**Technical Competence:** Being drawn to the content of work and being an expert in your field

**Discipline-focused:** Orienting toward structure, routine, and order

**Flexibility:** Adapting and "going with the flow." Here-and-now oriented

**Followership:** Taking instructions and directions and following them to stay on track

**Managerial Competence:** Managing a business unit and/or the work of others

**Self-directing:** Being guided by an inner compass

**Steadiness:** Working in a stable environment performing conventional, routine work

**Learning:** Continually studying and learning, intellectual activity

**Leadership:** Creating a vision, taking charge, and leading others to achieve results

**Accountability:** Doing what you say you will do and accepting responsibility

**Relating:** Building and maintaining genuine relationships. Finding deep satisfaction in working hard with friends to achieve a goal

**Connectivity:** Believing in the connectedness of everything and exploring interrelationships

**Visionary:** Creating a vision for the future and acting upon it

**Maximizing:** Maintaining an orientation toward the best in people, helping them to act upon it

**Restoring:** Bringing something back to its original design or intention

**Strategist:** Seeing patterns within things, concepts, and data. Generating alternative scenarios

**Artistic:** Creating through painting, acting, music, creative writing, computer graphics, and the like

**Creativity:** Creating something new, different, and helpful

## Instructions

Step 1: Review the 30 skill clusters and choose seven of them that best describe your key satisfying sets.

Step 2: Prioritize your seven clusters by imagining that you have been given $10,000 in the following amounts: one $3,000 bill, two $2,000 bills, two $1,000 bills, and two $500 bills. Write the amounts on your clusters accordingly, with $3,000 being given to your most often used, satisfying clusters.

Step 3: Decide, to the extent to which you are able, to use these skill clusters in your work. Write the word *green* on the sets that you almost always use in your current job, the word *yellow* on the sets that you can sometimes use in your current job, and the word *red* on the sets that you can hardly ever use in your current job. It is possible to have all one color on your seven sets.

## Transferable Skills Card Sort

The purpose of this exercise is to identify specific, key transferable skills that you enjoy using while working or during other times in your life. By transferable we mean that you can use them in a great variety of situations, as opposed to clinical or technical skills, which can be limited to a particular discipline.

You are given a list of 60 skills described on cards. On a piece of paper, draw five boxes and in them write the following information. As you review each of the 60 skills, write them under one of the five boxes.

| Totally Satisfying Skills | Very Satisfying Skills | Somewhat Satisfying Skills | Prefer Not To Use These Skills | Strongly Dislike These Skills |
|---|---|---|---|---|

However, you may have no more than **five** skills in the Totally Satisfying category. You may have less than five skills in this category, but attempt to identify at least three skills.

Remember that a Totally Satisfying Skill is something you can almost not not do. You probably use it in a variety of settings. Some people literally may get physically or emotionally sick if they cannot use their totally satisfying skills. You should be able to give many examples of how you use these skills.

You may have as many skills as desired in the other four categories. Your attention should be in maximizing the use of your totally satisfying skills and minimizing the use of strongly disliked skills. When forced to use them, some strategies for minimizing your disliked skills included:

1. Get a little better at it;
2. Design a support system;
3. Use your strongest skills to overwhelm your weaknesses;
4. Just stop doing it.

# Transferable Skills

### ALERTNESS
Being attentive and watchful of events, whether expected or unexpected, and responding appropriately

### SHAPE DISCRIMINATION
Seeing differences and contrasts in shapes, widths, and lengths

### PLANNING
Developing mission statements, goals, objectives, and action plans

### DIRECTING OTHERS
Managing, supervising, and telling others what to do

### SERVING
Attending to and responding to the requests and needs of others

### CALCULATING
Using basic arithmetic

### FLEXIBILITY
Accommodating others, using a variety of skills, and being prepared to change tasks frequently

### EFFICIENCY
Arranging activities to save time, money, or energy

### ASSEMBLING
Taking something apart and/or putting things back together (devices, puzzles, buildings, etc.)

### TOLERATING DISCOMFORT
Working in bothersome situations or awkward positions

### INNOVATING
Inventing, modernizing, transforming, and finding new uses for existing products or services

### SYNTHESIZING
Putting ideas and/or facts together in new, creative, and useful ways

### USING EXPERIENCE
Using past experience, training, or opinions to judge or evaluate people, things, or ideas

### USING FACTS
Using objective truth, reality, or knowledge to judge or evaluate people, things, or ideas

### BUDGETING/ESTIMATING
Planning financial needs and predicting the value, size, or cost of something

### RISK TAKING
Initiating activities that could lead to gain or loss

### DEPENDABILITY
Consistently performing required tasks or assignments according to quality standards

### DESIGNING/DRAWING
Creating plans for a new project, structure, or product, creating pictures

### DRIVE/TENACITY
Persistently working toward a goal, pushing yourself to do the best you can

### COOPERATING
Working with others to reach a common goal

### PERSUADING
Influencing the behavior or opinions of others

### DECISION MAKING
Taking action to accomplish something and taking responsibility for its consequences

### PERFORMING
Acting in a manner that illuminates, gives pleasure, or both

### AESTHETIC JUDGMENT
Using artistic abilities or sense of beauty to judge or evaluate people, things, or ideas

### TREATING
Undertaking a treatment to relieve physical or emotional problems

### USING CAUTION
Using care and discretion to avoid loss or injury

### POTENTIAL PROBLEM SOLVING
Anticipating future occurrences and acting to minimize their impact

### TOLERATING REPETITION
Duplicating activities, performing the same task or operation repeatedly

### WRITING
Producing meaningful and grammatical sentences and paragraphs

### EDITING
Correcting, proofreading, and revising written material for grammar, content, and style

### PRECISION/ DETAIL WORK
Working carefully and accurately, completing many different tasks

### FOLLOWING PROCEDURES
Completing tasks according to detailed guidelines and methodologies

### RECORD KEEPING
Keeping track of money, objects, or facts on written records

### CONVEYING EMOTIONS
Communicating feelings and causing others to appreciate or to feel them

### PRECISION
Completing work according to set limits, tolerances, or standards

### RESPONDING TO PRESSURE
Reacting to urgent situations rationally and calmly

### QUESTIONING
Devising questions that result in gathering useful information or reaching new insights

### NEGOTIATING
Arriving at mutually agreed upon decisions or solutions through discussion and give and take

### ANALYZING
Breaking a problem into its various components or basic elements

### ADVISING
Providing information or recommending solutions to others' problems

### RESPONDING TO FEEDBACK
Altering plans and actions based upon the input from others

### EMOTIONAL CONTROL
Remaining calm when others are angry or feel frustrated

*continued*

## Transferable Skills (*continued*)

| | | |
|---|---|---|
| **SORTING** Classifying, ordering, and ranking information or items | **STRUCTURING** Arranging, designing, formulating, and defining a system for people, things, or ideas, and putting them in order | **VERIFYING** Checking for accuracy, confirming and validating |
| **MOTOR COORDINATION** Moving several parts of your body together accurately and smoothly | **EXPLAINING** Giving advice to others, communicating information clearly and accurately | **UNDERSTANDING/TACT** Recognizing and/or responding to the feelings of others without offending or embarrassing |
| **INVESTIGATING** Systematically researching and gathering information | **RAPID REACTION** Responding quickly and appropriately to new or sudden events | **NUMERICAL REASONING** Using mathematical or statistical procedures to analyze data or solve problems |
| **CONFRONTING** Challenging others, telling them something they may not want to hear | **ENLISTING** Motivating people and gaining their support for a project or new endeavor | **VISUALIZING** Conceiving shapes or sounds, perceiving their patterns, and helping others to see them |
| **INITIATING** Starting new tasks, ideas, or projects | **TRAINING** Instructing people, conveying knowledge, and teaching new skills | **RESPONDING TO EMERGENCIES** Calmly and sensibly dealing with dangerous or threatening situations |
| **OPERATING/ADJUSTING** Operating machinery or vehicles or other equipment, making adjustments | **COUNTING/MEASURING** Checking items one by one, and determining length, angle, or weight | **STRENGTH/STAMINA** Performing heavy physical tasks or doing physically tiring work without becoming exhausted |
| **READING** Obtaining information from written material | | |

When you have completed this exercise, compare your specific, key, satisfying skills to your skill clusters. You should begin to see a pattern of talents and abilities. A third approach would be to identify personality strengths by completing the Myers-Briggs Type Indicator®. A free version of it called the Jung Typology test is available at www.humanmetrics.com. When you have identified your profile, read about it in a book entitled *Do What You Are* that relates your strengths to various careers.[11] The book should be available in many public libraries. Again, you should begin to see correlations between your Myers-Briggs Type, your skill clusters, and transferable skills, providing you with an enhanced sense of career direction and how you tend to care for yourself and others.

### Nursing Career Interests

Career development pioneers John Holland and Richard Bolles developed a model identifying six basic arenas of career interests. They are:

REALISTIC:  People who have athletic or mechanical ability, preferring to work with objects, machines, plants, and animals, or to be outdoors

CONVENTIONAL:  People who like to work with data, have clerical or numerical ability, work with detail, and follow instructions

SOCIAL: People who like to work with people to inform, enlighten, help, and heal

ENTERPRISING: People who like to manage, sell, persuade, and contribute to the bottom line

ARTISTIC: People who have artistic, innovating abilities, who like working in unstructured settings, using imagination and creativity

INVESTIGATIVE: People who like to observe, learn, investigate, evaluate, or solve problems.

## CAREER OPPORTUNITIES FOR NURSES[12]

| Area of Interest | General Skills | Career Opportunities |
| --- | --- | --- |
| Realistic | Motor coordination, manual dexterity skills | Surgery, dialysis, rehabilitation, hands-on training, equipment demonstration, technical product representation |
| Conventional | Data and repetition skills, numerical, financial skills | Cost analysis, financial administration, budgeting, policy coordination, regulatory compliance, OR scheduling, staff coordination, supplies and equipment management |
| Social | Communicating, instructing, guiding, serving, helping, human relations skills | Public relations, writing, counseling, direct patient care, staff education/training, educational consulting, health education advocacy, recruiting, rehabilitation, ethicist |
| Enterprising | Planning, leading, supervising, managing skills | First-line and middle management, nurse executive, committee leadership, project management, self-employment, nursing organization leadership |
| | Influencing, innovating, and persuading skills | Fund-raising, recruitment, internal organizational development, legislative work, purchasing, selling, marketing, inventing, mediating, patient advocacy |
| Artistic | Performing, writing, drawing, designing skills | Training, educational program development, creating journals and newsletters, art and music therapy, consulting to theater, TV, or film producers, writing articles, booklets, and pamphlets, computer graphics, promotional displays |
| Investigative | Researching, analyzing, systematizing skills, observational and learning skills | Nursing research, systems development, informatics, work process design, academic faculty, computer analyst, consultant, disease and infection control, security, human resource generalist (discrimination, employee relations, harassment) |

People generally express interests in two or three of these arenas. Which area of interest represents your first, second, and third choice? Form a three-letter code, such as SEA or ISC. To locate specific occupations associated with your three-letter code (not just healthcare related), consult the Dictionary of Holland Occupational Codes, Consulting Psychological Press. It should be in a public or college library.

# Strategies and Resources for Nurse Self-Care

What follows is a list of more than 35 strategies, resources, and tools gathered from interviews across the country and from our personal experience and research. Some can be easily implemented, while others require more time and energy.

The strategies are summarized in the middle column in the table on the following page. If your situation is similar to the description to the left of each strategy, you may wish to act upon that tactic. The personal benefit of doing so is described to the right of each strategy.

## Connect to Community

In recent years, Americans seem to be increasingly isolated from one another. This impression is more than subjective: it is borne out by the data. For instance, in his 2000 book *Bowling Alone*, sociologist Robert Putnam (2000) presented extensive data showing the ways in which Americans have become increasingly disconnected from family, friends, neighbors, colleagues, and our democratic structures.[13] And yet we are social creatures who need to connect with one another to find meaning and purpose in life. In community, each person brings an abundance of skills and experiences that create synergy (1 + 1 = 3). To support community building, we have created a small group facilitators guide available to pilot groups by e-mailing us at www.jlhenry.aol. For additional information on the relationship between soul, caring, and community, read the chapter on community in our book *Reclaiming Soul in Health Care* (1999).[14] Another resource is M. Scott Peck's book *The Different Drum: Community-Making and Peace* (1987).[15]

## Build Healthy Relationships

Make a list of the relationships in your life and sketch a diagram like the illustration on page 117. Identify key relationships by name and indicate whether they are generally positive (+) or negative (–) in the sense that you are having some problems with them. If possible and desired, develop some strategies to turn the negatives into

## Using the Strategies

| Your Potential Situation When you . . . | Strategy | Personal Benefits |
| --- | --- | --- |
| Feel isolated and experience limited intimate relationships | Connect to community | Support an unconditional positive regard from others |
| Remain in unhealthy relationships | Build healthy relationships | Accentuate the positive, minimize the negatives, resolve conflicts |
| Find that your self-knowledge and awareness of others is limited | Share your story | Connect to community; grow as a person and heal |
| Find yourself in a group needing purpose, structure, and dialogue | Call a circle | Enhance respectful conversation leading to resolution and/or action |
| Need to lighten up and appreciate colleagues | Visit "Nurses Are Angels" web site | Read about nurse-patient connections, humor, poetry, and the like |
| Desire to examine personal assumptions | Focus upon possibilities, not problems | Expand options and build resiliency |
| Lack clarification of staff and/or patient expectations | Explore the expectations of others and communicate your expectations | Improve understanding and avoid pitfalls |
| Place too much emphasis upon problems | Practice Appreciative Inquiry | Focus upon what is right with a person or group |
| Allow external events and forces to control you | Live your life with intentionality | Identify and focus upon informed values, choice,s and actions |
| Become too controlling, structured, and indifferent | Anchor yourself in the present moment | Experience self-, colleague-, and patient caring |
| Experience compassion fatigue and burnout | Care enough not to actively care | Set boundaries and know your limits |
| Stereotype | Practice the art of human complexity | Expand your appreciation of diversity |
| Become too serious and controlling | Laugh and engage in humor | Experience physical therapy and stress reduction |
| Develop rigid beliefs and assumptions about life/work | Live open-ended questions | Become more receptive to life/work guidance |
| Become closed-minded and unreceptive | Pray | Seek and receive wisdom and guidance |
| Experience stress and anxiety | Practice meditation | Invoke inner wisdom, depth, and peace |
| Are manipulated by cultural values and consumerism | Live simply | Enhance lifestyle, inner values, and money management |
| Perpetuate denial, blame, anger, and victimhood | Practice forgiveness | Let go of negative past events and experience life integration and learning |
| Find food and eating to be a disengaged necessity | Prepare food and eat soulfully | Appreciate the preparation, aroma, and taste of quality food |
| Experience detachment from nature caused by busyness and other distractions | Connect to nature | Enhance pleasure and the relationship between nature and spirituality |
| Feel lethargic and a loss of energy | Exercise | Improve physical, mental, and spiritual health |
| Become detached from people who share common interests and values | Join caring and holistically oriented healthcare associations | Participate in groups sharing a common sense of mission, values, and intentionality |
| Become self-absorbed and uncaring | Take a vow-of-kindness pledge | Active reciprocation of kindness with others |
| Experience the pressures of time, family, and work | Give yourself a Sabbath day and listen to music | Rest, relaxation, and pleasure. Find greater peace, balance, and harmony |
| Feel self-absorbed | Be present to others and listen | Live in the present moment |
| Engage in limited activities of self-care and have no self-care plan | Complete a self-care audit and develop a self-care plan | Evaluate one's current self-care situation. Set goals and make a self-care plan |

positives. You may wish to brainstorm such strategies with close friends. This exercise is good for solving conflicts and for building healthy relationships. It may also provide the motivation, whenever possible, to turn away from unhealthy ones.

Dad - Sally +    Eve -
Family    Work
Bill +    Boss +
You
Alice +    Alicia +
Beth + Leisure    Friends Bob -

## Share Your Story and Listen to the Stories of Others

The importance of storytelling can be seen in many arenas. In his book *The Healing Art of Storytelling*, Richard Stone (1996) takes the reader on an inward journey to relearn the healing art of storytelling. It includes step-by-step explanations of how we can use stories to uncover lost pieces of ourselves, discover places that are hidden wellsprings of healing, and satisfy the hunger for meaning in our lives. "Through storytelling we can come to know who we are in new and unforeseen ways. We can also reveal to others what is deepest in our hearts and, in the process, build bridges. The very act of sharing a story with another human being contradicts the extreme isolation that characterizes so many of our lives."[16] Storytelling represents a key strategy in terms of connecting to community and to soul. The following lists some specific tools to facilitate storytelling:

### OH Cards

OH Cards is a set of 88 picture cards and 88 word cards. You place the picture card on top of the word card and tell a story. The cards provoke sharing and insight, bringing to a conscious level many experiences in life. A total of 7,744 combinations are possible. The cards and instructions can be purchased from Eros Interactive Cards, 1-800-236-1683 or e-mail jocelyn@OH-Cards.com.

### A PBS Home Video on Everyday Spirituality

We highly recommend the use of a PBS Home Video featuring Thomas Moore entitled *Discovering Everyday Spirituality—Story*. It is divided into various segments, with Moore providing some background information followed by vignettes. Stop the video after each segment and involve your group in a discussion. For example, the first vignette is a mother describing to her little daughter the circumstances surrounding her birth. Group members would follow this by sharing stories regarding their earliest memories as a child. The video can be found at most public libraries, especially in larger communities. It may also be purchased via the Internet.

### A Book of Storytelling Starters

There exists an excellent resource book that may be used to facilitate story sharing for many hours, entitled *A Guide for Recalling and Telling Your Life Story* by Martha Pelaez and Paul Rothman, Hospice Foundation of America (1-800-854-3402).[17] It offers countless questions for personal reflection in terms of family, growing up, adult life, and growing older.

### A Book for Work Groups

Another resource, especially for work groups, is a book entitled *A Safe Place for Dangerous Truths: Using Dialogue to Overcome Fear and Distrust at Work* by Annette Simmons.[18] It deals with the "how-to" of creating genuine dialogue among people at work.

### Some Internet Sites

We recommend two resources on the Internet, the National Storytellers Network at www.storynet.org and Corporate Storytelling at www.corpstory.com. The latter describes Evelyn Clark's consulting business, Corporate Storytelling, and discusses capturing, authentic business stories and "walking the talk" in terms of marketing them.

### This Book

Ask group members to obtain a copy of this book, and then assign a specific nurse's story for each member to read for group discussion. What personal memories and experiences did it bring to mind? (For example, *"Diane's story about her cardiac patient reminds me of . . ."*)

## Call a Circle

Calling a circle is an ancient form of meeting that has gathered people into respectful conversation for thousands of years. Today, a modern methodology includes how to set an intention (mission, content), guidelines for opening and closing rituals, and how to promote receptive attitudes and guidelines for shared leadership. More information about the circle process is available on the Internet through a search engine such as www.google.com.

## Visit the "Nurses Are Angels" Web Site

For more stories about nurse-patient connections, visit this web site hosted by Christy Jones, RN, at www.nursesareangels.com. If you like, you can submit your own stories. The site also includes nursing poems, jokes, and sayings. Just a few of the nurse sayings are:

> Nurses call the shots;
> RN means real nice;
> Nurses are IV leaguers;
> Nurses can take the pressure.

## Focus upon Possibilities, Not Problems

In their book *The Art of Possibility*, Rosamund and Benjamin Zander (2000) claim that our perceptions of reality are invented. We enter the world hard-wired with certain assumptions based upon centuries of human experience.[19] Upon arrival and during the first few years of life, our mental "processors" are soft-wired with data from parents and significant others, assumptions about life and how it should be lived. But if it is all invented, rather than expending energy upon negativity and problems, the Zanders' suggest we may as well create a second universe of innovation and possibility. Two basic questions are given to help us make a paradigm shift: "What assumptions am I making that I'm not aware I'm making, that give me what I see?" and "What might I now invent that I haven't yet invented, that would give me other choices?" Those who continually challenge perceptions and assumptions and embrace potential are more likely to be resilient through times of change.

## Explore the Expectations of Others and Communicate Your Expectations

One simple, practical way to avoid the pitfalls of faulty assumptions involves exploring what people expect of you and communicating your expectations to patients, peers, and other staff members. These include expectations in terms of what they can anticipate from you and what you expect from them. This becomes especially critical for caregivers in order to avoid misinterpretation. Putting them in writing, when appropriate, makes them more concrete and available for review.

## Practice Appreciative Inquiry

Closely related to the art of possibility, Appreciative Inquiry (AI) challenges us to focus upon what is right with a person, group, or organizational system, as opposed to constantly searching for what might be wrong. According to its primary originator, Dr. David L. Cooperrider of Case Western Reserve University, AI asks us to pay special attention to "the best of the past and present" in order to "ignite the collective imagination of what might be." AI is about seeing that which others may not see. It heightens our awareness of the value, strength, and potential of others and ourselves and helps us overcome the limits that we impose, often unconsciously, on our own capacities. For additional information, visit www.appreciative-inquiry.org or obtain *The Thin Book of Appreciative Inquiry* (1998) (it is literally a thin book).[20]

## Live Your Life with Intentionality

Live your life with intentionality. Intentions help us to focus upon what is important and inform our choices and actions. Some examples from Jean Watson, PhD, RN, include:

- Honor nursing as the spiritual, spirit-filled practice that it is;
- Make an effort to "see" who the spirit-filled person is behind the patient or colleague;
- At the end of the day, offer gratitude for all.[21]

## Anchor Yourself in the Present Moment

Throughout history, philosophers have struggled attempting to understand and describe time. They probed whether time has a beginning, whether it has an objective feature, or whether it is only a product of subjective experience. Generally, before the nineteenth century, there was little or no perception of linear time. All time was viewed as circular, as in the seasons of nature. Linear time came about because of our attempts to measure it, causing many of us today to become fixated on *watch* time.

Based upon nursing research, we know that one of the key dynamics of caring relates to *being present* to oneself and others. In this sense, time serves as a way to evaluate whether one is truly being present. Time seems to speed up when we are truly caring; an hour seems like 10 minutes when we are engaged. On the other hand, when we remain detached and don't seem to care about a person or activity, time seems to drag. Think of a person you dislike who is dull or an argumentative know-it-all; in the presence of this person, 10 minutes may seem like an hour.

## Care Enough Not to Actively Care

When possible and appropriate, give yourself permission to be selective in your active caring. We can care for everyone by wishing the best for him or her. By active caring, we mean a direct presence and involvement. Even if it were possible, caring for everyone in this sense leads to unhealthy behaviors such as codependence. Caring promotes mutual empowerment of people. Codependent caring leads to compassion fatigue and burnout. An antidote to codependency is to care for oneself.

## Practice the Art of Human Complexity

At least some of the time, it is normal to stereotype and pigeonhole people, often in terms of first impressions. For this reason, it becomes vital to remember that, in re-

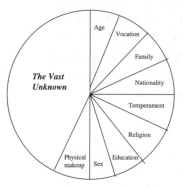

ality, humans are quite complex. We can be described by our age, what we do for work, our family background, nationality, psychological temperament, religion, education, our sex, and physical makeup.

Then, as many of us know, there resides within each of us a vast unknown. Whatever we call it—the unconscious (collective or singular), the shadow self, the "unused" portion of our brain—many psychologists think that it makes up the bulk of our psychological, spiritual, and cognitive makeup. Rainer Maria Rilke (1984) said, ". . . if we imagine this being (an) individual as a larger or smaller room, it is obvious that most people come to know only one corner of their room, one spot near the window, one narrow strip on which they keep walking back and forth."[22]

## Laugh and Engage Humor

Most of us know that laughter can be a form of therapy. Norman Cousins (1979) reminds us that "laughter is a form of internal jogging. It moves your internal organs around. It enhances respiration. It is an igniter of great expectations."[23] As a nurse, you can care for yourself and generate laughter by engaging a search engine such as www.google.com and typing, "nurse humor/laughter." Several sites are available.

In her account "Joe's Mom—A Story of Transformation," Lisa Wayman found it helpful to lighten up and have some fun in the midst of Joe's terminal illness. On the job, she sometimes laughs out loud at herself and makes jokes about some of the ICU equipment making dumb sounds. As it did for Lisa, humor helps us to not remain serious all the time.

## Live with Open-Ended Questions

In *Letters to a Young Poet,* Rainer Maria Rilke (1984) states, ". . . try to love the questions themselves as if they were locked rooms or books written in a very foreign language. Don't search for the answers, which could not be given to you now, because you would not be able to live them. And the point is, to live everything. Live the questions now. Perhaps then, someday far in the future, you will gradually, without even noticing it, live your way into the answer."[24] Living open-ended questions involves allowing the answers to come to you. It engages not a passive approach to life, but an active/receptive stance. For example, you might ask, "How am I to live the rest of my life? What is my destiny or calling?" We remain active during the ensuring days and weeks, but open to guidance from inner and outer voices of wisdom.

## Pray

In *The Soul of the Physician*, we shared that a significant number of physicians, as appropriate, pray either for or with some of their patients.[25] We approached this subject in the broadest sense, as described by Ann and Barry Ulanov in their book *Primary Speech* (1982). At the time of publication, Ann was a professor at Union Seminary in New York and Barry was a professor of English at Barnard College. They assert that, whether conscious of it or not, everyone prays, whether they know it or call it prayer. It is elemental discourse, such as pondering, "Why I am here." To pray is to seek wisdom and guidance. "We pray every time we ask for help, understanding, or strength, in or out of religion. . . . Our movements, stillness, the expressions on our faces, our tone of voice, our actions, what we dream and daydream, as well as what we actually put into words say who and what we are."[26]

As such, there is no best way to pray and there are no correct words to use. However, in his book *Healing Words* (1993), Larry Dossey, MD, suggests that a nondirective approach may be most suitable.[27] Here, we do not petition an outcome, such as telling God or the universe what to do. For example, as appropriate during career guidance sessions, Jim may suggest the following: "God (or your own metaphor), as you know, I am unhappy in my current job. I would like some guidance, and I am promising in advance to pay attention." The latter "paying attention" refers to the active/receptive stance. One might actively seek more satisfying work but be open to surprise and unexpected developments.

In a healthcare situation, a suggested stance might be simply to imagine a patient being surrounded by a shield of light. Or one might pray, "Your will be done."

## Practice Meditation

One physician we interviewed suggested that prayer involves asking, and meditation involves listening, or simply being mindful of an activity. As appropriate, home healthcare nurse Kathy Sitzman teaches patients to practice a walking meditation. They walk the perimeter of a room, counting the number of steps taken with each inhale and exhale of breath. It becomes a mantra, reminding us that life is workable if taken one step at a time, an easy method of reducing stress and anxiety.

Finding a still point in meditation—where busy mental activity subsides for a few moments—helps you to relieve stress and keep a clear head throughout the day.

- Sit comfortably with your back straight but relaxed;
- Close your eyes and become aware of your breath;
- Breathing normally, try to follow the inhalation and exhalation with your mind. Follow your breath, not your thoughts. Every time your mind is distracted by a thought, bring it back to the breath;
- Gradually you will feel the stress in your body and mind melt away and experience a deep, inner stillness and peace.

Another resource is a series of audiotapes by nurses Barbara Dossey, Lynn Keegan, and Cathie Guzzetta. Entitled *The Art of Caring* (1996), the tapes promote holistic healing using relaxation, imagery, music therapy, and touch.[28]

## Live Simply

Life simplification is about the movement away from consumerism, status seeking, and ego inflation to expanding choices and freedom. Through the Internet you can access any number of tips for prioritizing and simplifying your life. An excellent starting place involves examining one's life in relation to money. You might begin by reading Jacob Needleman's provocative book *Money and the Meaning of Life* (1991).[29]

Simplicity is not about poverty or deprivation. It is about discovering what is "enough" in your life—based upon thoughtful analysis of your lifestyle and values—and discarding the rest. The Skill Clusters Inventory in the section of this book entitled *Caring for Your Nursing Career* may also serve as a kind of values inventory and may help you to establish priorities.

## Practice Forgiveness

Because they often make life-impacting recommendations and decisions, healthcare providers especially need to practice forgiveness. It's been said that forgiveness involves letting go of the notion that you can change the past. The word is not limited to religious traditions. In fact, Harvard Medical School cosponsored a workshop on the subject of forgiveness. An excellent resource is a book by Suzanne Simon and Dr. Sydney Simon entitled *Forgiveness* (1991).[30] They remind us that forgiveness is a process, the end result of which is integration, wholeness, and learning. With respect to the latter, forgiveness is good for learning not to make the same mistake twice.

## Prepare Food and Eat Soulfully

In *The Re-Enchantment of Everyday Life* (1996), Thomas Moore reminds us that the "soul is not a mechanical problem that needs to be solved; it's a living being that has to be fed."[31] He suggests that food serves us in many ways. As we prepare it, we might meditate quietly. Its aroma is therapy. We taste food imaginatively. We find enchantment in its variety. A good cookbook can be an excellent source of earthy advice.

In addition, we highly recommend the cultivation of a garden, growing and caring for the earth and its bounty. It can serve as a place of meaningful toil, beauty, diversity, and contemplation, as well as rewarding your taste buds.

## Connect with Nature

Again, in *The Re-Enchantment of Everyday Life*, Thomas Moore treats us with an entire section on the relationship between nature and spirituality.[32] Much like a mother with her newborn child, nature will cuddle us in caring arms if we let it. It is so easy to be embraced by trees, rocks, streams and, above all, a household animal, such as a cat or dog. It is no wonder that often life-changing decisions are made during a retreat into nature. Moore challenges us to give up some of our busyness to enjoy it more often and to bring it into our homes and workspace, letting it care for the soul.

Even indoors, you can bring nature to your work environment by way of foliage and pictures of outdoor scenes, including the use of your computer screen. More and more, long-term healthcare facilities engage in this systematically through the Eden Alternative movement (www.edenalt.com).

## Exercise

Cardiac care nurse Diane Newman shared with us the importance of exercise as one of the main ways she takes care of herself. She loves to walk. She even joined a club in suburban Dallas walking with others about 10 miles every weekend. She especially enjoys walking in the early morning or at night, becoming one with surroundings. She also believes that if you can take control of your body, then you can be in control of other events in your life.

Some simple exercises that are good for you include:

- Walking 1.5 miles in 30 minutes;
- Bicycling 5 miles in 30 minutes;
- Swimming laps for 20 minutes;
- Gardening for 30 to 45 minutes; and
- Pushing a stroller 1.5 miles in 30 minutes.

## Join the International Association for Human Caring (IAHC)

The central purpose of the IAHC, Inc. is to serve as an international, scholarly forum for all nurses interested in the advancement of the knowledge of human care and caring within the discipline of nursing. Its core philosophy is based on the belief that caring is the essence of nursing, and caring is the unique and unifying focus of the profession. The association sponsors an annual conference and its web site is www.humancaring.org.

## Join the Relationship-Centered Care Network

Sponsored by The Fetzer Institute, Relationship-Centered Care (RCC) focuses upon ways to enhance and enrich relationships that are relevant to health care. The institute offers an excellent forum on their web site at www.fetzer.org/rcc/forum. The phrase "relationship-centered care" underlines that the relationship between people serves as the foundation for healing. As Colleen Person reminds us in the introduction to this book, health care in general, and especially nursing, must become a bio/psycho/ social/spiritual service.

## Participate in the Nurse Manifest Network

Nurse Manifest is a movement to awaken precious and powerful ideals that are rooted in nursing's worldwide historical traditions. They believe that it is possible to find connection in the midst of alienation, to find inspiration in the midst of cynicism, to find nourishment and meaning in the midst of spiritual impoverishment, and to find wholeness in the midst of fragmentation. The web site is www.nursemanifest.com.

## Explore Holistic Nursing

Holistic nursing requires that nurses integrate self-care and self-responsibility in their lives in order to help facilitate healing and caring for others. An interesting place to begin is www.dossey/dossey.com/barbara, the home page of Barbara Dossey, PhD, RN. Along with her husband, Larry, the Dosseys are trailblazers in holistic health care. Click on "A Conversation with Barbara Dossey." For example, she maintains, "Nurses can share and express their spirituality without using traditional religious language. Nurses can encourage their clients to explore the following reflective questions:

- What do I feel good about?
- With whom do I feel most free to 'be myself'?
- What is the hardest thing about my illness (or current dilemma) for my family and me?
- What helps me 'from within myself and from outside'?
- What worries me most?
- What am I afraid of?"

Another similar resource is a book by Dorothy L. Wilt and Carol J. Smucker entitled *Nursing the Spirit* (2001).[33] It includes a chapter on spirituality and holistic nursing.

## Take a Vow-of-Kindness Pledge

"I pledge to love my neighbor as myself and to make a difference in the lives of others. I pledge to do what I can to help bring about a kinder, gentler society, nation, and world." This is just part of the pledge suggested by the Acts of Kindness Organization, founded in Ohio and located at www.keepthekindnessgoing.org. The pledge helps us to be constantly on the look out for practical ways to show intentional kindness to others on a daily basis. Nonprofit, it was launched just after the September 11, 2001, tragedy. Along these lines, we recommend the book and movie *Pay It Forward*. It is the story about a junior high student who does a favor that really helps someone. He tells him not to pay it back, but to pay it forward to three other people who, in turn, each pay it forward to three more—and on and on into a global out pouring of kindness and decency.

## Give Yourself a Sabbath Day

The concept of resting on the Sabbath is not just for those of the Judeo-Christian tradition. It's solid advice for all of us, a day of rest from earning a livelihood and from routine work. What represents a favorite way to relax and enjoy yourself? If you are very busy, this might be a mini-Sabbath part of a day. You might also link this to meditation, music, relaxation techniques, and making a connection with nature.

## Listen

For most of us, listening is an obvious way to care for someone. Yet, during the busyness of work and life in general, we need to be reminded time and time again to slow down and listen to others and ourselves. Morton Kelsey (1981) captures the essence of listening as follows:[34]

| Types | Purpose | Examples |
|---|---|---|
| 1. Clarifying | To get at additional facts<br>To help her/him explore all sides of a problem/situation | "Can you clarify this?"<br>"Do you mean this?"<br>"Is this the situation as you see it? |
| 2. Restatement | To check our meaning and interpretation with her/his<br>To show you are listening and that you understand | "As I understand it then your plan is . . ."<br>"This is what you have decided to do and the reasons are . . ." |
| 3. Neutral | To convey that you are interested and listening<br>To encourage the other people to continue talking | "I see."<br>"Uh-huh."<br>"That's very interesting."<br>"I understand." |
| 4. Reflective | To show that you understand how he/she feels about what is being said<br>To help the person to evaluate and temper expressed feelings | "You feel that . . ."<br>"It was a shocking thing as you saw it."<br>"You felt you didn't get a fair shake." |
| 5. Summarizing | To bring all the discussion into focus in terms of a summary<br>To serve as a springboard for further discussion on a new aspect of the situation | "These are the key ideas you have expressed."<br>"If I understand how you feel about the situation . . ." |

## Listen to Music

Looking through the eyes of quantum physics, the elemental "stuff" or field of the universe is made of vibrating energy, which is also a way to describe music. Music serves as a universal language and healing force. It works to achieve balance and harmony, to integrate body, mind, and spirit.

Ronald Cole, MD (1998), reports a study about the positive impact of music at the University of Valencia. "One hundred and one babies [were provided] with taped violin sounds, arranged from simple to more complex forms, for up to 90 minutes per day beginning at about 28 weeks of gestation. Mothers exposed their babies to the music for an average total of 70 hours. At six months of age, the babies in the experimental group were significantly advanced in their motor skills, linguistic development, sensory coordination, and cognitive development when compared with controls."[35]

There are infinite possibilities relative to enjoying soulful music. Some that we particularly recommend include:

1. *The Geography of the Soul*
   The Chalice of Repose Project, Missoula, Montana, developed this music. This group works in hospice and palliative care, providing transitional music for those on the threshold of dying. However, the music is equally a resource for those in meditation entering a spiritual transition. Sapientia records, 1998.
2. *Transitions*
   Designed to sooth infants, this music combines a mother's heartbeat with natural harmonies. It is what an unborn infant might hear as mother listens to music. It is excellent for adults as well, but may conjure up strong emotions. Executive Producer: Fred Schwartz, MD, Plancenta Music Inc., 1987.
3. *DNA Music*
   This recording was created by Dr. David Deamer, an esteemed biologist at UCSC noted for his breakthrough work on the origins of life. He uses a technique called "mapping" to plot musical rhythms and combinations of tones that are charming and tuneful, as the bases proceed along the double helix. DNA Music creates a meditative mood. Available at New Leaf Distributing.

## Complete the Self-Care Audit[36]

We've been introducing the following self-care audit in some of our workshops, and people experience it as a real eye-opener. Few nurses or other healthcare professionals give themselves many "4s" and "5s," testifying to the reality that few of us take care of ourselves as well as we could. However, if this is your situation, don't let it depress you, but use it as a springboard for developing a self-care plan, which is the last strategy in this section.

## Self-Care Audit

Scale: Most of the time = 5  Some of the time = 3  Rarely = 1

| | |
|---|---|
| I share my joys, sorrows and disappointments with people I trust. | 5 4 3 2 1 |
| I do not compare myself with others by admiring or ignoring their gifts. | 5 4 3 2 1 |
| I have a small group of people I can call on for emotional support. | 5 4 3 2 1 |
| I take time to play. | 5 4 3 2 1 |
| I don't forget to laugh, especially at myself at times. | 5 4 3 2 1 |
| I often relax. | 5 4 3 2 1 |
| I protect my right to be human by not letting others put me on a pedestal. | 5 4 3 2 1 |
| I have learned to say no to unreasonable expectations, requests or demands. | 5 4 3 2 1 |
| I change jobs when I am miserable and pay attention to the things I enjoy in work. | 5 4 3 2 1 |
| I exercise. | 5 4 3 2 1 |
| I practice being a positive, encouraging person. | 5 4 3 2 1 |
| I pay attention to my spiritual life. | 5 4 3 2 1 |

## Develop a Self-Care Plan

Tom Ferguson, MD, offers the following worksheet for developing a self-care plan for your life:[37]

- My main area of interest (eating, exercise, learning to deal with common illness problems, etc.):
- My main personal strengths and resources in this area:
- The best resources for me in this area (people, groups, classes, books, etc.):
- Some activities and goals I might choose to help me explore this area (Brainstorm!):

- I would like to choose an initial activity that I could complete in about ___ days/weeks/months:
- Within this time limit, the goal I'd most like to set for myself is:
- Some small rewards I will give myself for making progress toward this goal:
- A big reward I will give myself for reaching my goal:
- The people I will ask for support in working toward this goal:
- I will contact my support persons on (date) to bring them up to date on my explorations in this area:
- My commitment, again, is to accomplish the following activities between now and the following date:
- On that date I will give my support person a report on my explorations in this area.

## Reflections on Caring: The Cycle of Self and Others

We began this book by postulating that many nursing professionals stand at the forefront in transforming the way health care is administered. We found this hypothesis affirmed, especially in terms of the intensive research taking place on the nature and processes of caring and its many practical applications.

Although Linda has an extensive background in healthcare education, communication, and marketing, neither of us is a nurse, which we believe was an asset. By looking objectively at the nursing profession from the outside, it allowed this book to be essentially written by and for nurses. We hardly scratched the surface of the two million-plus population of nurses in the United States, and certainly our intention was not to interview a random sample. Nonetheless, as Colleen Person testifies, many nurses today, like the phoenix, are beginning to rise from the ashes of the past to reclaim their unique professional caring relationships with patients and with one another. In today's technological, competitive, and results-oriented environment, more and more nurses are embracing creative mental, emotional, and spiritual ways to care. Individuals can make and are making a difference. And an increasing number of healthcare organizations are supporting these activities, encouraging self-care as well as the caring of others. They commit to this not only because of their value system, but also because of the reality that it makes good business sense.

One of Jim's mentors, Dr. Ruth Barnhouse, a wise and earthy psychiatrist and Episcopal priest before she died in 1999, used to say that there are only a limited number of ways to do bad things (she was undoubtedly thinking about the Ten Commandments), but an infinite number of ways to do good. We agree. In interviewing almost 30 nurses, we uncovered more than 100 strategies, resources, and tools for personal, patient, and organizational caring. Undoubtedly, many more exist and only time and publication constraints limited us in discovering them. We encourage our readers to continue expanding the list and sharing ideas with colleagues.

In the process of writing this book, we found a number of common themes:

▌ Many nurses enter the profession because of an innate desire to care and to make a difference;
▌ Many nurses view nursing as a calling;
▌ Creating a caring work environment makes a difference in turnover and staffing vacancy rate, and impacts patient and employee satisfaction.
▌ Creating a caring environment is not costly and has a positive effect on the bottom line.
▌ Self-caring begets caring. Nurses caring for themselves are key to caring for patients and colleagues, as demonstrated by the model shown below.

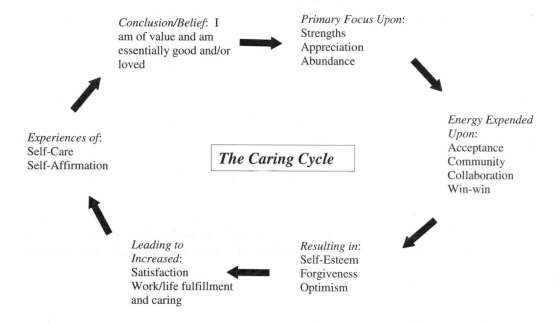

*Conclusion/Belief*: I am of value and am essentially good and/or loved

*Primary Focus Upon*: Strengths Appreciation Abundance

*Energy Expended Upon*: Acceptance Community Collaboration Win-win

**The Caring Cycle**

*Experiences of*: Self-Care Self-Affirmation

*Leading to Increased*: Satisfaction Work/life fulfillment and caring

*Resulting in*: Self-Esteem Forgiveness Optimism

As many nurses have told us, the transformative, caring cycle begins with self-care and affirmation. It leads to healthy conclusions and beliefs about oneself as being of fundamental worth and value. In turn, this leads to a primary focus upon strengths, appreciation of others, and upon abundance existing in the universe. Therefore, energy is expended upon acceptance, community, and collaboration, resulting in increased self-esteem, forgiveness, and optimism. The end result is increased fulfillment and caring, feeding back to and reinforcing self-care and affirmation.

Although remaining on this caring path is an ongoing challenge, the journey can be enormously satisfying. We encourage our readers to step on the path and invite people to share their personal experiences and resources for continuing this sacred journey with us at jlhenry@aol.com.

# Appendix
## Sample of Interview Questions

What early experiences led you to nursing as a career?

What does the word *soul* mean to you?

Describe a situation in your work when you experienced wonder and mystery.

Describe the characteristics of a nurse who is connected to soul/spirit.

What are you passionate about in your work (specifically related to Skill Clusters, Skills Card Sort, and MBTI® instruments)?

Can you describe a time in your nursing career when you felt deeply frustrated or disconnected?

What caused it? How did you cope with it and transition toward revitalization? In your own words, what do you think it means to be a caring nurse?

How are you implementing the processes of caring (as described by Dr. Swanson) in your work?

What keeps you in the healthcare profession?

After you die and at your memorial service, what would you hope your patients would say about you as a tribute?

What other (not caring-related) strategies and/or resources would you recommend to your colleagues in health care?

In what nonclinical ways do you develop yourself as a person? What do you read?

How do you enhance a sense of community in your life?

How have you dealt with a mistake you made?

There are those who say that the current healthcare climate of staffing shortages, time pressures, fiscal constraints, etc., prevents nurses from being caring individuals. How would you respond to that belief?

Can you share a humorous event in your nursing career?

Are you optimistic or pessimistic about the future of medicine?

Who are your heroes/heroines?

What are some ways a nurse can take care of himself or herself emotionally and spiritually?

# Notes

## Introduction

1. American Nurses Association, *Code of Ethics for Nurses with Interpretative Statements* (Washington, D.C.: American Nurses Publishing, 2001), p. 6.

2. American Nurses Association, *Nursing: Scope and Standards of Practice* (Washington, D.C.: nursesbooks.org, 2004), pp. 6, 12.

3. Jean Watson, the foremost scholar in caring theory, has her web page at www2.uchsc.edu/son/caring/content. It is an excellent first stop in learning more about caring theory in nursing. Madeleine Leininger's pioneering work as a nursing anthropologist led, among other things, to the formation of the Transcultural Nursing Society in 1974: http://www.tcns.org. Both scholars are also cited as key nursing theorists in *Nursing: Scope and Standards of Practice*, an essential reference on nursing practice (Washington, D.C.: nursesbooks.org, 2004, p. 12). See also Kristen Swanson's 1999 chapter, What Is Known About Caring in Nursing Science. A Literary Meta-Analysis. In A.S. Hinshaw, S. L. Feetham, and J.L.F. Shaver (Eds.), *Handbook of Clinical Nursing Research*. (Sage 1999), pp. 31–60.

4. Jacob Needleman, *The Way of the Physician* (New York: Harper Collins, 1985).

5. For further information on the Fetzer Institute, go to http://www.fetzer.org. To learn about the Magnet hospitals and their underlying Magnet Recognition Program™, go to http://nursingworld.org/ancc/magnet.html. For detailed and analytical background, consult *Magnet Hospitals Revisited: Attraction and Retention of Professional Nurses* (2002), by Margaret L. McClure and Ada Sue Hinshaw, available at http://nursingworld.org/books/. To find out more about Planetree facilities, start at http://www.planetree.org.

6. Kristen M. Swanson, Empirical development of a middle range theory of caring, *Nursing Research* 40, no. 3 (May/June 1991), pp. 161–166.

7. Bethel Ann Powers & Thomas R. Knapp, *A Dictionary of Nursing Theory and Research, Second Edition* (Thousand Oaks, CA: Sage Publications, 1995), pp. 1, 6.

## Part I

1. Diana J. Mason, Tell me a story—Knowing when and how to use nursing stories (editorial), *American Journal of Nursing* 103, no. 12 (December 2003), p. 7. http://www.nursingcenter.com/library/JournalArticle.aspArticle_ID=445295.

2. Marcus Buckingham and Curt Coffman, *First, Break All the Rules* (New York: Simon and Schuster, 1999).

3. Thomas Droege, *The Healing Presence* (San Francisco: Harper, 1992).

4. Mary Elizabeth O'Brien, *Spirituality in Nursing: Standing on Holy Ground* (Washington, D.C.: Catholic University of America Press, Second Edition, 2003).

5. Parker Palmer, *The Courage to Teach* (San Francisco: Jossey-Bass, 1999).

6. Cursillo is a Spanish word meaning "short course." The movement originated in Spain and was begun by Roman Catholics, but today is practiced worldwide and is also embraced by Protestant denominations including Methodists, Lutherans, and Episcopalians. Its purpose involves the deepening of Christian spirituality and community leading to authentic leadership and witness.

7. Carl Hammerschlag, MD, *Dancing Healers* (San Francisco: HarperSanFranciso, 1989).

8. Morton Kelsey, *Caring* (New York: Paulist Press, 1981).

## Part II

1. Kathleen Sanford, *Leading With Love* (Olalla, WA: Vashon Publishing, 1998).

2. *American Journal of Nursing*, 102, no. 106 (June 2002).

3. The Caring Model™ is a registered trademark and service mark of Sharon K. Dingman used under license.

4. See Implementing a caring model to improve patient satisfaction, *Journal of Nursing Administration* 29, no. 12 (December 1999).

5. Greg Levoy, *Callings: Finding and Following an Authentic Life* (New York: Harmony Books, 1997), p. 2.

6. James Hillman, *The Soul's Code* (New York: Random House, 1996).

7. Debra Farrington, *Hearing With the Heart* (San Francisco: Jossey-Bass, 2003), p. 76.

8. Martha Finney and Deborah Dasch, *Find Your Calling, Love Your Life* (New York: Simon & Schuster, 1998).

9. Linda S. Henry and James D. Henry, *The Soul of the Physician* (Chicago: AMA Press, 2002), p. 4.

10. Ibid., p. 200.

11. Paul Tieger and Barbara Barron-Tieger, *Do What You Are* (Little, Brown & Co, 1995).

12. Adapted from Bette Davis, *Career Planning for Nurses* (New York: Delmar Publishers, 1997).

13. Robert Putman, *Bowling Alone* (New York: Simon & Schuster, 2000).

14. Linda S. Henry and James D. Henry, *Reclaiming Soul in Health Care* (Chicago: AHA Press, 1999).

15. M. Scott Peck, *The Different Drum: Community-Making and Peace* (New York: Touchstone, 1987).

16. Richard Stone, *The Healing Art of Storytelling* (New York: Hyperion, 1996), p. 3.

17. Martha Pelaez and Paul Rothman, *A Guide for Recalling and Telling Your Life Story* (Washington, DC: Hospice Foundation of America, 2001).

18. Annette Simmons, *A Safe Place for Dangerous Truths: Using Dialogue to Overcome Fear and Distrust at Work* (New York: AMACOM, 1999).

19. Rosamund Zander and Benjamin Zander, *The Art of Possibility* (Boston: Harvard Business School Press, 2000).

20. Sue Annis Hammond, *The Thin Book of Appreciative Inquiry* (Plano, TX: Thin Book Publishing Company, 1998).

21. Jean Watson, Intentionality and caring-healing consciousness: A theory of transpersonal nursing, *Holistic Nursing Practice* 16 (July 2002), pp. 12–19.

22. Rainer Maria Rilke, *Letters to a Young Poet* (New York: Vintage Books, 1984), p. 90.

23. Norman Cousins, *Anatomy of an Illness* (New York: W. W. Norton, 1979).

24. Rilke, *Letters to a Young Poet*, pp. 34–35.

25. Linda S. Henry and James D. Henry, *The Soul of the Physician* (Chicago: AMA Press, 2002), p. 298.

26. Ann Ulanov and Barry Ulanov, *Primary Speech* (Atlanta: John Knox Press, 1982), p. 1.

27. Larry Dossey, *Healing Words* (San Francisco: HarperSanFrancisco, 1993).

28. Barbara Dossey, Lynn Keegan, and Cathie Guzzetta, *The Art of Caring* (Lewisville, CO: Sounds True, 1996).

29. Jacob Needleman, *Money and the Meaning of Life* (New York: Doubleday, 1991).

30. Suzanne Simon and Sydney Simon, *Forgiveness* (New York: Warner Books, 1991).

31. Thomas Moore, *The Re-Enchantment of Everyday Life* (New York: Harper Collins, 1996), p. 61.

32. Ibid., p. 6.

33. Dorothy L. Wilt and Carol J. Smucker, *Nursing the Spirit* (Washington, DC: American Nurses Publishing, 2001).

34. Morton Kelsey, *Caring* (Ramsey, NJ: Paulist Press, 1981), p. 77.

35. Ronald L. Cole, MD, *The Gentle Greeting* (Naperville, IL: Sourcebooks, 1998), p. 101.

36. Adapted from an audit on the Internet by Thomas Wright.

37. http://www.healthy.net/library/journal/self-carearchieves.

## Transformational Eldercare from the Inside Out: Strengths-Based Strategies for Caring

### James D. and Linda S. Henry

Created from interviews with nurses, educators, doctors, social workers, chaplains and long-term care administrators, this book and its companion Facilitator's Guide are designed to present a wide array of practical concepts, resources, and higher education and training programs which you can apply to your professional practice and/or your personal situation. Caregivers will learn about the nature of elderhood, not only in terms of growing problems and diminishment, but in promoting transformational elderhood as a time of life that is also marked by social, psychological, and spiritual expansion. The book contains more than 75 strategies and resources to enhance professional services and caring.

**Pub# 06TEIO**                         **List $34.95/ ANA Member $27.95**

## Transformational Eldercare from the Inside Out:
### Book and Facilitator's Guide

This easy-to-use facilitator guide is contained on a CD-ROM which can be used with the book. The instructor may adapt any parts of the materials in the guide to make it useful for his or her own training purposes. **The CD Facilitator's Guide is _not_ sold separately**

**Pub# 06TEIF**                         **List $49.95/ ANA Member $39.95**

## ORDER FORM

| Title | Price | Qty | Total |
|---|---|---|---|
| Transformational Eldercare from the Inside Out   (book only) | | | |
| - - - - - - - - - - - - - - - - - - - - -  Book & Facilitator's Guide | - - - - - - - - | - - - - - - - - | - - - - - - - |
| Shipping & Handling | | | |
| TOTAL | | | |

### Shipping and Handling

| | U.S. | Outside U.S. |
|---|---|---|
| Up to $25 | $4 | $8 |
| $25.01-$50 | $6 | $12 |
| $50.01-$100 | $8 | $16 |
| $100.01-$200 | $14 | $24 |
| $200.01-$300 | $12 | $32 |
| $300.01+ | 7% of total | 15% of total |

**Payment:** (Payment in U.S. dollars required)
[  ] Check enclosed (Made payable to Nursesbooks.org)
Charge my [  ] VISA      [  ] MasterCard

Card # _____ Exp Date _____

Phone _____

Signature _____

**Ship to:**

Name _____

Organization _____

Address _____

_____

City/State/Zip _____

**Nursesbooks.org, P.O. Box 931895, Atlanta, GA 31193-1895, USA**
**Phone: 1-800-637-0323   Online: WWW.NURSESBOOKS.ORG**